I Don't Know What to Eat

The Definitive Guide to Food Allergies, Intolerances, and Sensitivities
and What to Do About Them

By Helen Adams

I

Get Helen's FREE webinar: How to deal with food intolerances:

https://www.oakmeadclinic.co.uk/i-dont-know-what-to-eat/

Join the Facebook group 'Nutrition on a Plate'

Get your FREE ECOURSE with 21 days of recipes by typing this link into your browser: https://www.oakmeadclinic.co.uk/digestive-rescue-in-just-21-days/

Author: Helen Adams

Title: I Don't Know What to Eat

Subtitle: The Definitive Guide to Food Allergies, Intolerances, and Sensitivities and What to Do About Them

Subjects: Food and drink; diets and healthy eating; healthy eating

To all my clients,

*whose countless questions
inspired me to write this book.*

Acknowledgements

So many people have provided input into this book, sometimes knowingly and sometimes not. My thanks are due to all my clients whose simplest questions have sometimes caused me to dive into research for hours on end to be able to answer the most basic: "How?" and "Why?" I always wanted to add on: "What next?"

My thanks are also due to all my colleagues, fellow-kinesiologists and nutritional therapists who enthusiastically joined in with suggestions of things they would like to know so that my clinic wall was covered with post-it notes of all the things I needed to include in this book.

During the months of writing, I canvassed opinion from anyone who would listen because everyone is an expert on food; we learn about it throughout our lives, and our real experiences are often worth so much more than just a theory on paper.

Finally, every author should have a solid review team behind them. My husband, Wilf, brought his technical authoring skills to bear in fine-tuning the detail and making sure it said what I thought I had said. My children also made their thoughts known in a few areas concerning presentation and getting the point across, and many enthusiastic supporters helped with general purpose reviews to make sure it flowed well and made sense.

My thanks to one and all, I couldn't have done it without you.

A Few Words from My Clients

"I've seen other nutritionists who have very set ideas and restricted my diet. This made me quite stressed as I like eating out and couldn't find anything on a menu that I could eat! Helen has a completely different approach, she actually listened and offered solutions which really related to my needs & were sensible. My condition is much improved after only 3 sessions. Helen is very approachable & easy to get on with, highly recommended." MW, Upper Westwood

"Thank you so much for all your help. I've lost inches from my waistline, my energy has returned, my brain fog has lifted, and I feel fantastic. What made the difference wasn't just telling me what foods were causing me problems, but telling me how to plan and shop for replacements, and how to get organised so I had the right things in the house. All my family and friends are asking me what I've been doing as the difference is so obvious. I will be sending them all to you!" EJ, Chippenham

"I'm now much more aware of my food choices for myself and my family. During my weekly shopping trips, you are never far from my thoughts." KS, Bath

"I was unsure what nutritional therapy would do for me and initially was sceptical. I began to improve and am now able to track the link between foods and symptoms. Helen has helped me to understand how I can manage my diet and well-being in a way that works." KS, Bristol.

Contents

Who Should Read This Book?

Food is our friend - or so we are told. Food is fuel, and we need to consume enough fuel to power us. However, how much thought do we give to that fuel and the way it works? Using food wrongly can be like putting the wrong fuel into a high-performance sports car: the engine won't perform properly and, eventually, it will just give out. Every day of the week I meet people who have problems with food. Their issues range from a minor irritation to a crisis which has a severe impact on the way they feel and restricts the things they can do. They don't understand the cause, so they give it the label 'allergy' because they feel so terrible.

They may have a 'food baby' after lunch and know they can't wear tight clothes that won't allow for a severely expanding waistline. They may navigate their day by reference to toilet locations and how long it takes to travel between each one, just in case they get caught short. They may have put up with severe headaches and pains for years, not realising that the cause is constipation that can be made many times worse just by certain foods. If you remove these foods from your diet, then the body's natural detox improves. The symptoms disappear. In some cases these food problems have lasted for years, gradually getting worse, but people don't understand the causes or what to do about them.

There are many food bloggers out there offering solutions. Some are very well qualified, some aren't, but to the layperson, the distinction isn't always obvious. There is a mountain of conflicting information in the public domain suggesting this diet or that, depending on the latest fad. It's tough to pick your way through this minefield when all you know is that something doesn't feel right. Many of my clients begin their consultation with: "This is probably wrong but…" or worse: "I had a food intolerance test a year ago, and the practitioner told me that I was intolerant to twenty-five foods. I've excluded all of them since then, but I don't feel any better…" They need help.

You'll find that this book is a little different: I've not shied away from being controversial here and there, but I've tried to explain the reasons behind that. I passionately believe that the tools for good health are there, in front of us, if only we could recognise them. We just need to keep an open mind, to be willing to make small changes and to try something new. Yes, it might mean having to make a bit more effort in the kitchen. No, I'm not suggesting spending hours slaving over long lists of ingredients you've never heard of to make something inedible that goes straight in the bin (I've been there!). You might have to do some planning to make sure you have the right foods in the house to start with, but it's all doable. Most of all, it just means having the courage and desire to take the first step and to move on from there.

Are you with me...?

This book is for you if:

- You suspect certain foods make you feel unwell, whether or not you can identify which foods are the culprits;

- You are confused by the difference between an allergy, a sensitivity, and an intolerance (and what difference do the terms make when you can't eat it!);

- You discussed your symptoms with your doctor, who told you that you don't have an allergy and that there is no such thing as a food intolerance;

- You had a food intolerance test, but the follow-up didn't tell you how to interpret the results, so you avoided all the problematic foods and found your diet too restrictive;

- You had a food intolerance test, but you didn't understand what to do next - so many things came up - so you quietly put the report in a drawer and forgot about it;

- You are thinking about getting a food intolerance test, but don't know how to go about it or which one to pick;

- You've already done quite a bit of reading about food and food intolerances but want to do more research before you make any decisions.

How to Use This Book

We are all different, and sometimes it can be difficult to understand why someone else who seems to eat the same things that you do seems to be in excellent health while you feel tired, listless or moody. You may have irritable bowel syndrome (IBS) or skin problems or struggle to lose weight. I want to explain the reasons for this:

Part I covers the difference between food allergies, food intolerances, and food sensitivities. You'll also find explanations for situations that may present themselves as a food allergy when they're something entirely different (for example Coeliac disease, which is an autoimmune disease).

Part II is all about the foods and allergens (these are foods that cause undesirable reactions). The Top 14 allergens are discussed, as well as many familiar food groups that cause intolerances and sensitivities. If you want to know about any food group, just head to the contents pages to find out where it's in the book. You'll also see that I've included what is right about these foods as well as their nutritional profile. I don't agree with excluding many foods from your diet just on the basis of a food test (though you might exclude a subset of foods as a *temporary* measure until you get your body back to better form).

The best health comes from a full diet with lots of variety. That way you don't have to work out whether you've enough of any vitamin or mineral, you are going to be getting what you need. Lots of variety has added benefits for your population of friendly gut bacteria as well – if they thrive, in return, they support your health in a mutually beneficial relationship. If you exclude foods, you *must* replace them with something else, and I provide suggestions. Maintaining the diversity of your diet can support the overall balance of your body.

I include some science to explain what happens when you have food issues. All these sections are signposted with 'The Science behind....' I know some people will want to dive into these and others will quite happily skip over them. You'll still find plenty of interesting and useful information, whether you are scientific or not.

Understanding food labelling is essential for anyone with food issues. I've included the regulations and alternative names to look out for so that your 'old enemy' doesn't slip back into your diet through the back door.

You'll soon see that severe allergens have the same list of possible reactions, severe intolerances have a similar list, and there are lots of groupings of foods, either by botanical family or because they have a chemical compound in common. In some cases, problems arise because the body gets confused between similar-looking chemicals and reacts to them in the same way, or because of previous exposure to something else. It can be quite a complicated picture. There's plenty of information here to help clarify matters, but some people will just say: "I'll get a test."

Part III covers all sorts of testing, not just the narrowest definition of food intolerance testing, although of course that's covered. I've included what is available on the NHS and what isn't, and what the tests are measuring. Not everyone wants to be tested, and not everyone needs to be. If you do take a test, you'll be taking it with full knowledge of the advantages and disadvantages of the different types that are available.

Part IV is all about solutions. The solutions aren't limited to just "cut out 26 foods," as one of my clients was previously told. Good health must start from within, so there are recommendations on simple measures to start that journey. Getting these things right will go a long way towards resolving so many issues. My Top Tips are also here to help you do this for yourself.

Part V gives you some helpful resources that I refer to throughout the book. They include some self-help tools so you can be fully involved in this voyage of discovery. Even better, I've added free downloadable copies of my self-help tools on my website for anything you need to fill in. Just look on www.oakmeadclinic.co.uk/free-stuff/ to find them.

The book includes references for those who want to find the appropriate studies.

Throughout the book, the terms 'practitioner' and 'therapist' are interchangeable, as are 'he' and 'she.'

This book is all about food: some of those foods will be things that many people know they can't eat now, like tomatoes or peppers. If you already know (or suspect) you have a problem with that food then exercise caution with my suggestions. My suggestions are just that and aren't intended to suit everyone. (For example, if you have a nightshade sensitivity then celery is a good substitute for bell peppers, but if you are allergic to celery then you shouldn't eat it). You can always contact me for more specific recommendations for your situation.

At the end of the book, I've included chapters on useful online resources and a little more about the therapies I use to provide greater context.

Aims

This book aims to show you that our relationship with food has many aspects. Understanding what lies behind unpleasant symptoms is part of the answer, but there are many solutions available which are neither difficult nor expensive to implement.

There are triggers in our environment that make food issues more likely, such as pollution and toxicity affecting the food, reduction in nutrients due to soil depletion or just poor food choices.

The answer isn't to exclude every problematic food, which just creates more illness, but to heal the body so that many problem foods can be eaten once more.

Additionally, I give my advice in the debate of whether to test or not test for food intolerances and discuss alternatives. There is no one size fits all solution to food issues. Everyone's journey is unique, and this book will allow you to recognise alternatives and decide on the right path for you, guided by extensive knowledge. Knowing helps you feel in control of your health, and when you have that control, you'll achieve a much better outcome.

My website details are below; there you can find further information about free resources, my services and how to contact me.

https://www.oakmeadclinic.co.uk

My Story

I'm a healthcare practitioner. As you would expect from someone in my profession, I'm very healthy, but this wasn't always the case. My family history is one of strokes, cardiovascular disease and cancer. I had eleven surgical operations and fell into the category of 'never well since' a bout of Epstein-Barr virus when I was eighteen years old. That kept me away from school for most of the year. I always had a positive outlook, so I just thought it was 'normal' to have frequent health problems. I thought they were an inconvenience and carried on with my busy life. When my son was born, things changed.

He was premature, had significant digestive issues since birth and by the age of ten was severely ill. He was small for his age and for a whole year he didn't grow at all. He spent months away from school. Finally, the consultant diagnosed chronic fatigue syndrome. "At last!," I thought, "we will get some treatment." Unfortunately, this wasn't the case. There is no magic drug to make things better for chronic fatigue syndrome. The only thing on offer was a graded exercise programme; it was a coping mechanism to avoid energy burnout. It was a tough sell to a young child desperate to do what all the other children did, and the best I can say is that it didn't work for him.

I wasn't content to accept that there were no other solutions, and so I started to look at various therapies outside our National Health Service (NHS). Identifying food intolerances seemed to be a crucial part of many therapies, and at one stage my son was told to avoid all gluten, dairy, yeast, and sugar due to food intolerances. There was a long list of other banned foods, and we duly tried our best to stick rigidly to the exclusions. No-one told us about introducing any other substitutes, so, of course, his diet became even more restricted and different to that of the rest of the family and his friends. Can you imagine how difficult that was, seeing us eating all the things he would like to eat when he was barred from touching any of them?

He also hated vegetables and wouldn't eat anything green, so our choices were quite limited. I often felt that the practical element was missing from practitioners' advice. How could it be possible to avoid all those foods and live on such a restricted diet? If he didn't keep to it, how severe would the consequences be? How would we know which omissions were the key ones? We didn't have the answers to those questions. It was all or nothing. Everyone found it complicated. Now when clients tell me their stories of how they tried to get better by eliminating many foods from their diet I can empathise with their experience.

At that time there was no gluten-free aisle in the supermarket, the concept of online shopping was only just starting, and there were very few easily available raw ingredients to use as alternatives. I've always hated cooking, but after a long working week, I was in the kitchen all day Saturday, every week, trying to make gluten-free food that was edible. I used to make bread from an Australian packet mix, heavily based on corn. It crumbled almost immediately it came out of the oven, and it was edible for just a day. I tried various types of bread, but they were very dense – very far removed from the light and fluffy offerings in the shops. I used xanthan gum to give them some 'lift,' but this often leaves an aftertaste. Many of my 'creations' just went straight in the bin. It was all costly, very time-consuming and I had no idea how to manage such a massive problem with food.

A breakthrough came when we discovered an excellent nutritional therapist. She arranged lab tests, gave us recipes and a dietary supplement regime. Just as importantly she 'held our hands' and guided us as things changed with my son's health. The lab tests showed that it was taking three days for my son to create energy from a meal. It was no surprise that he was so tired. The tank was empty!

The turning point for me was when she suggested eating a red pepper every day. It's a bright colour (not the hated green), very juicy and sweet-tasting yet packed full of vitamins and nutrients. There is more vitamin C in a red pepper than there is in an orange. Very gradually things started to change, and I became hugely enthusiastic about nutrition (though still entirely clueless in the kitchen, I will admit). I was explaining the latest test and treatment to my hairdresser one day when she said, "You know so much about this subject, why don't you become a practitioner yourself?" It was as if a lightning bolt had hit me and instantly my mind was made up.

As soon as she left, I researched what I would need to do to qualify as a nutritional therapist. Now I was hungry for formal training to fill in the gaps in my knowledge and to teach me many new things about how the body works (and what to do about problems).

Throughout my son's journey, I became acutely aware of the strengths and weaknesses inherent in the different therapies we tried. My most significant frustration was that, although there was something to be gained from all of them, they weren't joined up. They each seemed to exist in an isolated bubble and I wanted to ensure that my therapeutic offering didn't fall into the same trap.

I became a full-time student, entirely focused on learning. I believe there is never just one answer to improving health. We are all individual and different approaches work for each of us, so I wanted my learning to cover a wide range of possibilities. I learned about anatomy and physiology – what makes the body and how it works. I took a three-year nutrition diploma with the College of Naturopathic Medicine (CNM) to learn how to nourish the body with food. I also spent three years learning kinesiology to diploma level. Kinesiology equipped me to look at the body's energetic imbalances and the interplay with the emotions. It includes structural techniques as it originated from chiropractic. Kinesiology gives me a way of testing just about anything, and it's quick, easy and painless to carry out.

I came across iridology as a diagnostic tool and completed a postgraduate diploma in that. Iridology tells me about health dispositions inherited from each parent, plus of course many issues acquired during a person's lifetime. Several more years followed studying functional medicine, with its emphasis on the whole body rather than individual symptoms and the patient's timeline to see when issues began and the sequence of ill-health since then. Functional medicine also makes good use of appropriate lab testing to delve deeply into areas of concern and stresses using food as the first form of medication before drugs.

Although the approach of each 'discipline' seems to have very significant differences at first glance, particularly between naturopathic and functional and scientific and energetic, there are common threads that run through them, and I've included more information about them at the back of the book for those who want to know more. I quite happily hop between these different approaches in my clinic, depending on what will be most beneficial for the client. The fundamental principles aren't that different, and I do refer to many of them in various ways in this book – and encourage you to do some detective work yourself using some of the techniques!

As for my son, at the time of writing this book he's a university student. He now plays sport, enjoys long walks in the countryside and still has enough energy for other hobbies. He no longer has chronic fatigue. He always avoids gluten but he can eat anything else, and he does eat many vegetables!

Caveats

I'm not a medical doctor; I'm a qualified nutritional therapist, a functional medicine practitioner and a kinesiologist. This book has been written for general information and not to diagnose or treat any illness. Much of the information I describe here can be used to improve your wellbeing, but should you be at all concerned about the possibility of any medical condition you should see your doctor. Seeing your doctor is crucial if you've had any symptoms of pain or bleeding from the rectum.

If you are already experiencing a serious health condition and you are under the care of a specialist, he may prefer you not to make any changes to your diet in case this disturbs your drug regime in any way. We don't become ill due to a lack of medication but due to a lack of nourishment – here, I mean nourishment in its broadest sense. Not just food nourishment but also the emotional nourishment that comes from a sense of community and belonging.

The right diet can make a significant difference to your health, and it's always worth exploring how food can help you, but you don't need to do this alone; use the guidance of a competent practitioner. Their years of training can fill in the gaps in your knowledge and ensure that your medication and food are working together to support you, not against each other.

Emotions can affect any part of our bodies and remain hidden for years as unseen baggage. It's when I'm constructing a Functional Medicine Timeline with someone, or using a kinesiology technique that gets to the same issue, that there is an "Oh my God…" moment. They realise their problems with foods began in childhood when their parents were divorced; the cat died; they moved house or any number of other events that had a profound significance for them.

In adulthood relationships at work and home can sometimes be less than ideal, and your body responds accordingly. Some people already understand that emotions can have a significant impact on the body. For those more logical people who don't think that's relevant, this book has much science too; all I ask is that you are open-minded about all of it, even if sections of it don't agree with your belief system.

Just as there are many ways that illness can happen, there are many ways to restore health. Medications are designed to address one symptom, which is why you can end up taking several drugs - each with a different purpose - and sometimes more medicines to deal with the side-effects caused by the others. They don't deal with the cause of illness, and you can end up taking them for a lifetime. As soon as you stop, the symptoms return. By December 2014, almost half the women and 43% of men in England were regularly taking prescription drugs [1]. Attending to your 'nourishment' in its fullest sense can make such a massive difference to your health that many drugs may no longer be required – but medicines have potent effects on the body, and you should always discuss any changes to the dosage with your doctor. Withdrawal from some drugs can give you rebound symptoms that are as bad or worse than the original health problem.

Part I: Food Allergies, Intolerances, and Sensitivities

How Do You Know if You have an Allergy?

If you think you may be allergic to something and don't know what it is, you should start to keep a record of your symptoms – use the Food Allergen Identifier in the Helpful Resources chapter. You can also download a usable copy of this for free from my website, www.oakmeadclinic.co.uk/free-stuff/

You can also use these questions to help you:

- Do you only get symptoms at particular times of the day?

- Do your symptoms occur at certain times of the year?

- Are your symptoms more noticeable during the day?

- Are your symptoms more noticeable during the night?

- Do your symptoms occur when you are inside the house as well as outside?

- Does exposure to animals bring on your symptoms?

- Do you think that any particular food or drink brings on your symptoms?

- Do the symptoms occur every time you encounter the allergen?

- Do your symptoms improve when you are on holiday? [2].

Definitions

> *"According to Allergy UK, only 2% of the population suffer from food allergy, but an enormous 45% of the population suffers from some type of food intolerance."*

These definitions may help you understand whether you might have an allergy, an intolerance or a sensitivity. I set out the definitions of these terms in more detail a little later, but, for the moment, here is an overview. These conditions aren't characterised by symptoms but by the biochemical mechanism that creates them. Some of the difficulties of working out which definition applies to you arise because the symptoms can seem so similar across the three groups. However, what *causes* those symptoms is entirely different. Understanding the cause helps to inform the possible solution.

There is a considerable difference between the naturopathic and functional medicine schools of thought, on the one hand, and the western medicine tradition (your GP and the NHS) on the other. There is a place for both. The naturopathic and functional medicine schools are looking at the whole person: what has made them ill and restoring balance to the entire body. Western medicine is looking at an individual symptom or organ where dysfunction reaches the level of disease. When there is a disease, the doctor will usually prescribe a drug to manage the symptom. He may prescribe a second medication to control the side-effects of the first medication.

With my training in naturopathic nutrition and functional medicine, I always want to know *why* something is happening.

- A **food allergy** is an immediate immune response to food. This immune response can be life-threatening

- A **food intolerance** is a non-immune reaction to food. This response can be rapid, but not usually life-threatening

- A **food sensitivity** is a delayed immune response to food. It isn't life-threatening and can take up to three days to appear.

Please note that in the public imagination the terms food intolerance and food sensitivity are often regarded as the same thing, when they have entirely different causes, as explained above. It's helpful to know the difference between all three definitions so that you can form a better idea of what to do next and understand how the different approaches that I outline can deal with the various problems. Intolerances and sensitivities can also result in very vague symptoms that are hard to pinpoint and only seem to occur some of the time. This can be a quantity issue.

Allergy Symptoms

Allergies cause a reaction, within 2 hours or less, that primarily affects the skin, airways, and digestive system. You don't even have to eat the food – sometimes the smallest particle in the air, or a touch on the skin, is enough. Children's allergies may disappear with time. Allergies that occur as an adult are usually lifelong [3]. Some allergies can result in such an extreme reaction that it can be life-threatening, but this isn't the case for all allergies. You could develop an allergy to any food if your family have allergies or allergic diseases, such as asthma or eczema. If both of your parents have allergies, you are more likely to develop a food allergy than someone with only one parent who has allergies [4].

Food Intolerance Symptoms

Food intolerances occur because the food needs a substance to break it down – usually an enzyme (a substance that breaks down other proteins that aren't required anymore, keeping everything working as it should) - and your body isn't making that enzyme. A food intolerance is nothing to do with your immune system and therefore doesn't involve antibodies (antibodies are cells that your immune system creates to respond to a foreign invader).

Just because a food reaction has a significant impact on your health and lifestyle doesn't mean it's an allergy. Food intolerance reactions can occur rapidly (within hours, but not as suddenly as allergies) as your body reacts when it's trying to break down the food you've eaten.

In some cases, you don't make the enzyme because you don't have enough of the raw materials to be able to do so. Change your diet to include the raw materials (more protein), and you could see a difference. In other cases, your body doesn't make the enzyme because it's considered unnecessary (or no longer necessary, as happens with lactase, the enzyme that breaks down the sugar in milk).

The reactions you would see from intolerances are flushing, cold or flu-like symptoms, inflammation, diarrhoea, and general discomfort [5].

Typical foods in this category are lactose, sulphites, histamines, lectins, preservatives, artificial colours, fillers, flavourings, chocolate, citrus fruits, and acidic foods.

Food Sensitivity Symptoms

Food sensitivities are a widespread problem. Ten people could eat the same foods and experience ten different immune responses, all due to food sensitivity. There is no 'one size fits all.' There is a kinesiology saying: "where it is, it isn't," which means that symptoms are found in a different place to the cause of the problem, and this is undoubtedly the case here.

Food sensitivities are one of the most challenging areas to pinpoint, as there could be (and usually are) multiple sensitivities involved and it can take as long as seventy-two hours after eating the food for symptoms to appear. Symptoms can affect any part of the body.

The symptoms could be any of the following:

> Fatigue or hyperactivity, headaches or migraines, dizziness, muscle or joint pain, digestive issues – irritable bowels, bloating, constipation, diarrhoea, nausea, vomiting, or indigestion. There can be difficulty sleeping, food cravings, skin problems – excessive sweating, acne, rashes, hives, dry skin, bladder control issues, unintentional weight loss or weight gain. There can also be dark circles under the eyes, runny nose, sinus problems or ear infections, mood swings, anxiety or depression, asthma or wheezing, or irregular heartbeat.

Typical sources of food sensitivities are the proteins in milk (cow's milk, goat's milk or sheep's milk and their products such as cheese or yoghurt), eggs, gluten from several grains (not just wheat), soy, shellfish, and tree nuts. Any food could become a sensitivity.

If you have any food sensitivity, it's more than likely that you have more than one. People are often dismayed to find they have issues with so many foods, but I always stress that foods should be taken out of the diet with care and replaced with something else to at least maintain, and possibly increase, diversity in the diet. The good news is that food sensitivities can be resolved over time so you'll probably be able to eat many of these foods in the future (there is more information about individual foods in the following chapters).

Meet Some of My Clients

Some of my clients have stories to tell:

Sue

Here is Sue. She has a food intolerance:

Sue is very active and is a keen runner. She has a busy job involving much walking. She's always rushing to the next thing and eats her food 'on the go' most of the time. Her weekly treat is to stop in the local coffee shop and have a cake and a latte. Unfortunately, she can guarantee that virtually every time she has her treat in the coffee shop, she needs a sudden trip to the bathroom. Occasionally she doesn't make it in time, and this can be very embarrassing. Sue reacts to the lactose in the milk that goes into her latte.

Lactose is a natural sugar that needs a specific enzyme, lactase, to break it down. Many people stop producing lactase at around the age of two – lactose breaks down breast milk, and when we start eating solid food we no longer need to drink milk.

In some cultures, such as the Far East where they don't drink cow's milk, it's normal to be intolerant to lactose. In the West, dairy milk has become so much part of our culture for generations that there is now a genetic mutation that means people continue to make the lactase enzyme (so *many* people can drink cow's milk – but probably not *all* people).

Martina

Let me introduce you to another of my clients, Martina. She has a food sensitivity:

Martina wanted some help with weight loss and fatigue. When I first met her, she looked as if she had had quite a few late nights recently, with dark rings under her eyes. Martina looked pregnant, even though she wasn't. She tried sporadic calorie restriction to lose weight, but it left her hungry, tired and miserable whenever she did it. The weight never seemed to go. She wasn't dieting at the time but still felt constantly fatigued. She suspected something she was eating might be causing her swollen stomach.

She had tried to identify it herself but could never pin it down. Martina just knew that sometimes she felt a little better and sometimes a little worse, although she was always tired. She was also constipated, managing to go to the toilet only once every two or three days. She had some reflux and took over the counter medications for that. Martina felt quite miserable because everything she did seemed almost too much effort and she couldn't remember a time when she didn't feel this way.

Martina has a sensitivity to gluten, found in the bread that she craves.

Pauline

Pauline has a food allergy:

She experienced a very dramatic trip to the hospital as a child. She was at a birthday party when her throat started to feel very itchy. Her mother noticed she was constantly trying to clear her throat. She was coughing, then wheezing. Within minutes the wheezing got worse. She stopped playing and was having difficulty breathing. She started to feel very light-headed. Fortunately, Pauline was very close to the hospital, and her mother took her there straight away. Her airways were closing due to an allergic reaction.

It was less than half an hour since she had eaten a small crumb of peanut. The doctor gave her an injection of adrenaline (also called epinephrine in the US). Adrenaline calms the immune reaction that caused the allergic response (more on that a little later).

Ever since that time she carries an 'EpiPen' in her handbag, keeps another in her car and one in her desk at work, just in case. An 'EpiPen' carries a shot of adrenaline that she injects straight into her thigh at the first sign of any contact with a peanut. This area of the body is rich in blood vessels, which are the body's superhighway network to transport all manner of substances around the body.

Adrenaline is rapidly transported 'systemically' (all around the body) to calm the generalised inflammation that closes the airway and causes other issues too. Pauline doesn't even have to eat a peanut to be affected; just a trace amount which she breathes through the air or on her skin will be sufficient. She has had to use her 'EpiPen' a few times since her original diagnosis. She also wears a 'MedicAlert' bracelet to alert others to the cause of her problem, should she be unable to inject herself in time.

Anaphylaxis is the name of this very severe, life-threatening type of allergy. Not every allergy will be this severe, but the main points to note about food allergies are that they cause immediate reactions – occurring within anything from just a few minutes to half an hour of eating or encountering the food, but certainly within two hours. Even trace amounts can be enough to cause the reaction.

You might sometimes have been on a plane where they have announced that no peanuts are available because someone on the plane has a peanut allergy and has asked that no-one consumes nuts. Allergic reactions are the extremely rapid onset of rashes or hives, obstruction of the airways (wheezing and difficulty breathing), itchiness of the mouth and problems with the digestive system (often diarrhoea).

Why Do Food Allergies Occur?

Surveys show that as many as 30-35% of people worldwide could be affected by allergies at some stage in their lives [6]. Between 1990 and 2007 UK hospital admissions for anaphylaxis (an extreme, life-threatening reaction where the airways close) rose by 700%, and for food allergies by 500%. Prescriptions dispensed for all types of allergy have increased since 1991 [7]. No-one knows for sure why food allergies are so much more common although there are several theories:

One view is that we are just 'too clean.' This theory is known as the 'hygiene hypothesis.' In previous generations, children played outside in the dirt and encountered the local environment with all its germs. They developed a tolerance to their surroundings that made their immune systems much less active. 'Oral tolerance' is tolerance to things that first enter the body in small quantities through the mouth.

Think of children with dirty hands and babies putting everything in their mouths, be it toys or food or anything else they happen to pick up. I can just about remember making mud pies in the garden as a child. Without electronic gadgets, everything we explored was a potential toy.

Nowadays children spend much more time indoors, living in sterile environments. There is a more significant toxic load due to increases in dust mite populations in centrally-heated, draught-free homes, and we wipe away every trace of germs with strong chemicals. We don't let children get dirty. We bathe them frequently at just the age they should be exploring the environment outside. Such cleanliness changes the way our immune systems work and instead of keeping us safe, as all the marketing would suggest, the lack of constant exposure to new microbes means we react more strongly when we encounter new things. There is growing evidence that the way a person first encounters a food has a bearing on whether an allergy will develop. People can become sensitised (build up an allergy) if the contact is through the skin (breathing in tiny particles or touching the food). If people eat the food, they develop a tolerance to it - this means the immune system doesn't see that food as a threat [8].

A research paper in 2016 suggested that eating a high fibre diet including vitamin A could reduce the incidence of allergies by developing several different mechanisms in the gut to promote greater oral tolerance [9]. Fibre-rich foods are fruit and vegetables and legumes (beans). If we encouraged the consumption of these foods from an early age, perhaps we would see fewer allergies develop.

Another possible reason for increases in allergies is to do with diet. Previous generations ate local, seasonal food that was fresh. They had more variety throughout the year because each season had different fruit and vegetables that weren't available at other times. In turn, this increased the diversity of bacteria in their gut (our gut bacteria can be quite fussy – they like certain foods, and if we don't feed them, they reduce in numbers).

The healthiest people have the most diverse gut bacteria – the diversity helps us digest more food and supports our immune system [10]. Although now we have access to most fruit and vegetables at any time of year, we don't necessarily choose to vary them and often eat the same vegetables from one week to the next.

Many people eat a very restricted range of vegetables, despite the abundant varieties that are available in the shops. Foods that aren't seasonal could have a long journey to get to the store. Many are harvested before they're fully ripe and finish ripening on the journey or even in the store. Picking them before they're ripe reduces the nutrient content. Lower quantities of nutrients mean less support for the immune system. Good health includes developing an appropriate immune response (more on this later).

We have become quite obsessive about exposure to sunlight. UV light is by far the best mechanism for generating vitamin D, which is essential to develop the tolerance we need in the immune system [11]. In certain latitudes (including the UK) it's difficult to get enough exposure to UV rays from the sun to generate sufficient vitamin D between October and early March [11] [12].

Add to this our modern lifestyle, with more office-based and indoor working, and the government health messages to use copious amounts of high-factor sun cream and sunblock when we are outside. The result is that many people have low levels of vitamin D (with consequent impact on their immune system).

We should be aware of the risks of skin cancer. However, we need to strike the right balance. We are now seeing the return of terrible

20

diseases like rickets in children whose skin is never exposed to the sun without sunblock [12] [13].

The most common food allergies in children are to milk and eggs, but fortunately, these often resolve before adulthood as 'Oral Tolerance' (mentioned above) retrains the immune system. Oral tolerance is where the immune system recognises that food proteins you've eaten aren't threats to your health after all and so the immune response that causes allergies and sensitivities is weakened or suppressed. This suppression occurs throughout the body (this is called 'systemic'). In effect, the army 'stands down' [14].

In adults, most allergies are to cow's milk, eggs, wheat, soy, peanuts, tree nuts, fish and shellfish.

Food Allergies in More Depth

The Science Behind Food Allergies

I've tried to keep the technical explanations within the science sections. If you aren't interested in science, you can just skip these parts, and you'll still get a lot out of this book. If you would love to learn what allergens and antibodies are and how they work, then read on.

Protein is one of the major food groups that our bodies need; it's the building block that supplies raw materials for our DNA to make other things, on demand. It builds connective tissues like the skin and muscles as well as hair and blood. You may have seen 'protein powders' in some health food shops: bodybuilders use these to increase their muscle bulk rapidly and repair the damage caused to tissues from making those muscles work very hard. We don't just get protein from powders though; we should always look to food first.

Proteins have a role to play in maintenance and repair: they make enzymes. Proteins also make up your immune system, so you see that protein is an essential part of our diets. The immune system consists of a network of cells, tissues and organs that work together to protect the body from invaders. There are many different cells in the immune system, and they each have specific jobs to do. These cells patrol the

21

parts of the body that are in contact with the outside world - the gastrointestinal tract, nose, mouth and skin. They also patrol the inside of the body. Immune cells called antibodies are involved in food reactions.

If your body identifies a harmless food particle as a threat, it creates antibodies to deal with that threat. That results in an allergic reaction, and the food particle (a protein) becomes an allergen. There are five types of antibodies, each with a different chemical structure while having the same recognisable shape - they look like a letter 'Y.' They can identify different allergens with the 'arms' of the 'Y,' but the immune system always recognises the stem.

Recognition is important because your body is a world, with different continents and different cities as well as transport links – from superhighways down to small tracks impassable by vehicles, and different populations. The immune system must be able to recognise what is 'self' and what is 'non-self' to function correctly (when this distinction becomes garbled, autoimmunity ensues).

The type of antibody responsible for allergic reactions is IgE (Immunoglobulin E), which accounts for only 0.002% of the total antibodies in the blood. Almost all IgE antibodies are attached to cells called mast cells and eosinophils. When we talk about an IgE allergic response, it's called 'IgE-mediated.' You'll see this term often mentioned in this book, mediated just means 'related to IgE.'

Mast cells are white blood cells found in the membranes lining the nose and just under the surface of the skin. They're in the eyes, skin, respiratory tract and intestines too. They release histamine. Histamine causes inflammation, with which you'll be very familiar in terms of itchy and puffy eyes, runny nose or possibly a blistering rash (think hay fever). Inflammation occurs on the inside of the body as well as on the outside, and the danger comes when that inflammation causes the throat and the airways to close, making it hard to breathe.

Inflammation pumps more fluid into all the spaces in the body that are 'under attack,' thus making more room for the immune cells to move around, replicate (make exact copies of themselves) and flood the area with chemical messages that attract even more immune cells to come and fight. When the airways close the person may become weak and floppy and may have a sense of something terrible about to happen. They may collapse and fall into unconsciousness. The fact that you can't breathe is collateral damage and your immune system – like any good army - is wholly focused on killing the enemy, whatever that takes.

Your body makes the different cells in the immune system according to need. Eosinophils usually make up a tiny part of your immune system but, in response to an allergic reaction, the levels can increase up to 5% of all immune cells. They live in your blood, and they're attracted to inflamed tissues. Here they release more inflammatory chemicals. They're measured when your doctor takes a standard blood test: a raised level of eosinophils is a sign that your body is fighting an infection or parasites.

IgE antibodies detect the invaders and amplify the immune response by calling in other types of immune cell, like calling in reinforcements. IgE-mediated reactions are also responsible for allergic reactions on the skin or in the airways such as hives, asthma, and hay fever [15]. Anti-histamine is usually the treatment for minor to moderate food allergies [16].

The Science Behind the EpiPen – How it Works to Control Anaphylaxis

EpiPens contain adrenaline (epinephrine), which is a hormone made by your adrenal glands (hormones are chemical regulatory messengers that move around the body to deliver instructions to the cells with which they interact). Adrenaline prepares the body for 'fight or flight' by acting on the walls of blood vessels, causing them to tighten. Blood pressure increases. Adrenaline also works in the heart and lungs to make the heart beat stronger and faster and to relax and open the airways. The overall effect of all these things is to increase the amount of oxygen in the blood, which is transported to the muscles and tissues to ready them for action. It also prevents the release of further allergic chemicals, thus reversing the action of histamine [17] [18].

Food-Dependent Exercise-Induced Anaphylaxis

Anaphylaxis is a rare form of allergic reaction that occurs when a combination of factors is present. There are usually specific foods (more than one) that could be allergens, together with exercise. The foods in themselves don't cause an allergic reaction, and the activity on its own doesn't cause an allergic reaction. Put both those factors together, and suddenly there is a very severe reaction that could result in an emergency hospital trip to treat an acute anaphylactic response [19].

There are a few theories as to how this might happen: it might relate to the increased speed and quantity of histamine release under exercise conditions. It could be due to the increased blood flow to muscles and away from the gut (which means the immune cells would be travelling around the body faster and more efficiently) [20]. More research is needed.

Potential foods involved in food-dependent exercise-induced anaphylaxis could be wheat, shellfish, nuts, tomatoes, peanuts, fish, pork, beef, mushrooms, hazelnuts, eggs, peaches, apples, milk or alcohol [20].

Allergens and Food Labelling

An allergen is a substance that causes an allergic reaction [21]. The Food Information for Consumers Regulation (EU) No. 1169/2011, updated in December 2014, states that foods sold non-packed or prepacked for direct sale must provide allergen information. The allergens are now highlighted in bold text in the list of ingredients to make them easier to see.

Manufacturers must use advisory warnings if their products may contain one of the fourteen allergens through accidental contamination. This unintentional contamination could arise at any stage from growing the ingredients (for example, rotating crops in a field, or transporting sacks of grain in a truck which has also previously transported wheat) to processing the ingredients in a factory that also processes one of the allergens.

Manufacturers often use the warnings as a safeguard, to protect themselves in case there could be any contamination.

Examples of advisory warnings:

- May contain [xxx]

- Made with equipment that also processes [xxx]

- Made in a factory that also handles [xxx].

[xxx] is the name of the 'top 14 allergen' that could contaminate the food. These warnings are highly important, but they don't tell you the impact of eating the allergen.

The Top 14 Allergens

The top 14 allergens, as described in the legislation, are:

- Cereals containing gluten, namely wheat (such as spelt and Khorasan wheat), rye, barley, oats and their hybridised strains and products thereof. Except: a) wheat based glucose syrups including dextrose b) wheat based maltodextrins c) glucose syrups based on barley d) cereals used for making alcoholic distillates including ethyl alcohol of agricultural origin

- Crustaceans and crustacean products (for example prawns, lobster, crabs and crayfish)

- Egg and egg products

- Fish and products thereof, except a) fish gelatine used as carrier for vitamin or carotenoid preparations; b) fish gelatine or Isinglass used as a fining agent in beer and wine

- Peanuts and peanut products

- Soybeans and soybean products, except a) fully refined soybean oil and fat; b) Natural mixed tocopherols (E306), natural D-alpha tocopherols, natural D-alpha tocopherol acetate and natural D-alpha tocopherol succinate from soybean sources; c) Vegetable oils derived phytosterols and phytosterol esters from soybean sources; d) Plant stanol ester produced from vegetable oil sterols from soybean sources

- Milk and milk products (including lactose), except: a) whey used for making alcoholic distillates including ethyl alcohol of agricultural origin; b) lactitol

- Nuts (namely almond, hazelnut, walnut, cashew, pecan nut, Brazil nut, pistachio nut and Macadamia nut (Queensland nut)) and products thereof except for nuts used for making alcoholic distillates including ethyl alcohol of agricultural origin

- Celery and celery products

- Mustard and mustard products

- Sesame seeds and sesame products

- Sulphur dioxide and sulphites at concentrations of more than 10mg/kg or 10mg/L (litre) in terms of the total SO2 which are to be calculated for products as proposed ready for consumption or as reconstituted according to the instructions of the manufacturers

- Lupin and lupin products

- Molluscs and mollusc products (for example mussels, clams, oysters, scallops, snails and squid).

"The use of icons or symbols to indicate the presence of allergens is permitted. It must be accompanied by words and numbers to ensure uniform consumer understanding and to avoid misleading the consumer. Currently, there is no single agreed set of icons or symbols across Europe for indicating the presence of allergens in prepacked and non-prepacked foods [22]."

Accidental contamination is possible when you are eating out. For example, it's common practice to wipe a wok between dishes as the high cooking temperatures involved will kill any germs - but this doesn't remove traces of allergens. It's also possible that the food you are allergic to could accidentally get into another dish if the kitchen staff use the same serving spoons or utensils for different plates [23].

Allergies only require the tiniest amount of allergen to cause immediate reactions that could be severe enough to need an EpiPen. Using separate spoons or pans could be vitally important for some people. Those with food intolerances or sensitivities can eat a small amount of the problem food without triggering a significant response, and the scenario above wouldn't cause an issue.

Nuts and Food Labelling

Food labels aren't required to distinguish between 'nuts' (meaning tree nuts) and 'peanuts.' Tree nut allergies and peanut allergies are two separate allergies. If someone has an allergy to peanuts, he won't necessarily have an allergy to tree nuts and vice versa. The lack of clarity in the labelling can result in people avoiding both types of nuts unnecessarily when they only have an allergy to one of them [24].

Oats and Food Labelling

Oats don't contain gluten; they include a similar protein called avenin. It's possible that oats may be contaminated with gluten (see section on oats). According to the legislation, food manufacturers must include oats in the category of 'grains that contain gluten,' (as you'll see in the list of the Top 14 Allergens above,) because of the cross-contamination risk.

Another feature of the legislation is that (according to the food manufacturer Mornflake) if manufacturers were to sell oats made up into porridge using the instructions on the packets then the product would be allowed to be sold as 'Gluten Free' [25]. You may see products on the supermarket shelves labelled gluten-free and some others that aren't marked gluten-free, where the only difference is in the packaging and not in the oats themselves.

Food Sensitivities in More Depth

How Do Food Sensitivities Affect the Body?

Symptoms are just your body's way of telling you something is wrong. In kinesiology, we know that when you don't feel well, the body is in a state of 'imbalance'. Kinesiology uses the Chinese acupuncture energy meridians. In both kinesiology and acupuncture, the meridians are all connected; one flows into the next so that too little energy in one meridian will result in too much energy in another (there is always the same amount of energy altogether, but it may not be distributed correctly). Now we have a problem in at least two places.

The longer the original problem is there, the more imbalances could develop. As more imbalances develop, they present more symptoms. In kinesiology, there is a technique called 'clearing compensations' which removes all the 'sticking plasters' that your body has invented to try to deal with the original problem. Your body is continually trying to keep you in good health. The 'clearing compensations' technique is like taking a layer (or several layers) off the problem. It makes it easier to see what is going on underneath. The kinesiologist knows then that what they're working on is the priority problem.

Functional medicine also wants to get to the root of the issue, rather than just fix a symptom. According to functional medicine, one condition could have many different causes and, likewise, one cause may result in many different conditions. We certainly see this with all the food issues, whether they're allergies, food intolerances or food sensitivities because the symptoms are so similar that symptoms alone aren't enough to differentiate the cause.

Naturopathy looks for the 'rule of three': three pieces of evidence that support the hypothesis. These pieces of evidence could be symptoms, medical history and tests (tests don't have to be lab tests. A test could be as simple as eating some of the suspected food to see what happens next). The best tool to unravel the client history is the functional medicine timeline. The timeline looks back to when the problems began. There's no doubt that food sensitivities can have a huge impact, but is it any wonder that they can be so difficult to pin down when it seems that almost any food can produce a multitude of symptoms?

28

One of my clients, Gillian, is a pastry chef. All day long she makes terrific cakes for people. As part of her work she often tastes her creations to make sure they're just right for her customers. Gillian came to see me for a food intolerance test because she was having uncomfortable digestive symptoms, including what appeared to be random tummy pains, constipation and brain fog. In her mid-twenties, she thought she was too young to be ill!

She saw her doctor, but he said there was nothing wrong with her. I took her case history and did some testing. It turned out that she was sensitive to gluten and I recommended that she exclude this from her diet for a month to see what difference it would make. When I saw her again, I couldn't believe the difference. All her symptoms had gone, and she was feeling so much better. Nowadays she still makes cakes containing gluten, but leaves the tasting to others!

The Science Behind Food Sensitivities

I've explained previously that Immunoglobulin E (IgE) is the antibody associated with allergies (this is the antibody that doctors test for). Sensitivities result in a different antibody reaction involving the antibody called IgG (Immunoglobulin G). IgG is the antibody that's present in the highest quantity in your body, making up 80% of the total antibodies and 75% of the antibodies found in your blood.

IgG is the only antibody that can pass through the walls of small blood vessels to detect allergens in the spaces of the body outside the blood vessels. It's also the antibody which gives protection to babies for the first six to twelve months of life, derived from the mother's immunity passed on through the placenta. The baby's immune system matures during the first six to twelve months of life and can then function on its own. IgG antibodies are particularly useful for attacking extracellular viruses and pathogens [15].

The Role of Alcohol in Food Sensitivities

While we may enjoy a glass of wine on social occasions, and we are aware of its immediate effects on the body, we are a lot less knowledgeable about the effects of alcohol that lead to food sensitivities.

The gut is 'the outside on the inside.' It's a hollow tube running right through the body with exposure to the outside world at both ends. As far as the rest of your body is concerned, it's a danger zone that needs to be very well protected to keep invaders away. The gut is so important that there are three mechanisms to provide this protection. If anyone of those mechanisms is impaired, there is still some level of protection from the other mechanisms.

First, the gut has a thick layer of mucus on the surface closest to food (the inside of the tube). It's protective because it makes it difficult for invaders to penetrate. Secondly, there are microbes in between that protective mucus layer and the thin tissue that lines the gut (called the epithelium). These bacteria keep the surface of the tube sterile, which in turn protects it from some types of damage. Thirdly, the epithelium itself is made up of cells that are tightly joined together at their junctions. These tight junctions prevent any invaders getting through into the inside of the body. These junctions are the last line of defence against the invaders. These three protective measures are all active at the same time. Nutrients break down into very small particles that are small enough to flow through the various barriers and into the body to nourish it.

Alcohol disrupts the integrity of the gut barrier by breaking the tight junctions between the cells [26]. This means that it's easier for particles of food proteins to enter the body and trigger an IgG-mediated immune response (the immune response is triggered only by proteins, not by other food groups such as carbohydrates or fats).

Alcohol affects the bacterial population by causing inflammation in the gut. The bacterial community is significant as there are some species of bacteria that support us (we'll call them 'friendly bacteria') and other species that are pathogens. They don't help us at all. Inflammation kills off the friendly bacteria. Binge drinking can be particularly damaging as the friendly bacteria don't recover during the period of abstinence in between binges. Please take note, all those people who know they drink too much on the weekends and think this is safe because they don't drink during the week – it isn't [27].

What can you do about this? If you have several food sensitivities and you drink alcohol, this could be adding to your issues. The only answer is to stop drinking for four to six weeks to allow your body time to recover and to let those three defence mechanisms build back up to full strength. If you drink heavily, it may be easier to reduce gradually. Doing this alongside the other measures discussed in Part IV: Solutions could make a big difference not only in preventing new sensitivities from occurring but also in healing the ones you already have. If you want to start drinking again after that time, just do it in moderation.

Food Intolerances in More Depth

When we start to look at food intolerances – reactions that aren't caused by the immune system – we uncover a great many reasons why you and your food may not have such a great relationship. The good news here is that with a little knowledge, and some careful detective work, you can identify these reasons and do something about them. If you suffer from any food issues, I strongly recommend that you start to keep a detailed food diary. Write down everything you eat and drink, including the quantities and the times you eat. Write down your symptoms and when they occur (how long after eating).

Eating is one of the most fundamental processes of life, and as such we don't give it much thought. In my experience, most people have to think hard to remember everything that they ate today and certainly don't remember everything that they ate yesterday.

As I learned at CNM, one of the roles of the practitioner is to be an educator – to help the client understand the reasons behind their symptoms and, by doing so, give them back control of their health. With that in mind, we will look at the stomach and work out what's going on there.

The Science behind Food Intolerances – Stomach Acid

We all know we have stomach acid. It's ten times more acidic than lemon juice, and it has many important jobs to do:

- It helps break down food into small particles for digestive enzymes to continue the process. An enzyme is something that facilitates other chemical reactions. Digestive enzymes speed up the rate at which proteins in your food are broken down;

- Everything in the body happens within a pH range (a specific range of acidity or alkalinity). Enzymes are no different, and stomach acid provides the correct pH for those enzymes to work;

- Let me introduce you to pepsinogen. It's an inactive enzyme produced by specialised cells in the stomach called chief cells. What is the point of creating an inactive enzyme? It's a protective measure to avoid damage to the chief cells. There is a thick layer of mucus between these cells and the inside surface of the stomach. Acid can't penetrate the mucus; when the inactive enzyme meets stomach acid on the other side of the mucus layer, it's converted into its active form, pepsin. It can then break down proteins without fear of unintended damage to your body;

- Stomach acid destroys invading microorganisms that have entered your body through your mouth.

In case you were wondering why stomach acid doesn't dissolve your stomach, its chemical predecessor is produced in specialised cells (called parietal cells) in an inactive form, just like pepsinogen. It only becomes active through another chemical reaction that takes place when it reaches the other side of the mucus layer, where it causes no harm to your body [28].

How is food broken down in the stomach? The stomach is just a big bag that has muscle fibres running across it in different directions. The muscle fibres contract to churn the contents of the stomach in various ways and move stomach acid through the food, just like the action of a washing machine pushing washing liquid through the clothes and lifting out the dirt. In the same way, just as clothes won't get clean if you don't add enough of the active agent (the washing liquid), the food in your stomach can't break down sufficiently well if you don't have enough stomach acid.

Insufficient stomach acid could be due to medication such as proton pump inhibitors (shortened to PPIs). You may have heard of omeprazole (Prilosec) and lansoprazole (prevacid), which are designed to reduce the amount of stomach acid you produce to protect the oesophagus (the food pipe between your mouth and your stomach). This protection may be needed for various medical conditions such as gastric reflux, ulcers, and Barrett's oesophagus.

Sometimes doctors prescribe PPIs for acid reflux. There are other medications called H2 antagonists that also reduce the level of stomach acid, such as ranitidine – this is now available over the counter from pharmacies and supermarkets. PPIs prevent damage to the cells above and below the stomach that don't have natural protection from acid. In the case of Barrett's oesophagus, this damage could develop into cancer.

Any amount of acid causes damage to the throat. Medications are treatments that deal with one symptom. Unfortunately, they have downstream consequences if you take them for any length of time (more on this below).

Time for a recap. You don't have enough stomach acid, and you are still getting symptoms of gastric reflux? How does that happen?

One of the concepts of functional medicine is that many symptoms could have one cause, and many causes could have one symptom. In this case, stomach acid travels out of your stomach into your oesophagus and burns it. There are many possible causes:

- Your diet has low protein. Protein breaks down into individual amino acids and then reassembles into whatever your body needs 'on demand'. Cells are made, broken down, and made again as required on a continuous basis. If you don't take in enough of the raw materials, your body can't create the new elements needed to function – that applies to stomach acid and digestive enzymes too;

- Protein imbalances: good protein sources are cheese, eggs, fish, legumes (these foods have seeds in pods, like peas), meat, nuts and seeds, soy, and yoghurt. In the West, our meals tend to be protein-light for breakfast and lunch and protein-heavy for our evening meal. It's better to spread protein throughout the day - make sure each meal contains some protein;

- Sphincter incompetence: there is a sphincter at the top of the stomach. It's a ring of muscle that opens to let food into the stomach and closes to keep it there. Researchers have known since 1995 that there is a strong association between reflux and 'incompetence' of this sphincter ('incompetence' is a medical term which means it opens when it shouldn't) [29]. These events are brief and intermittent rather than the sphincter being persistently defective. The sphincter relaxes due to foods like alcohol, chocolate, citrus, coffee and other caffeinated beverages, fatty foods, garlic, onions, peppermint, spearmint, tomatoes, and whole milk [30] [31]. If you eat or drink any of these, there is the potential for a small amount of stomach acid to exit the stomach and splash back up into your oesophagus. You can check out these foods yourself and see if they're related to your symptoms;

- Infection by a bacterium called Helicobacter Pylori (sometimes called H. Pylori). Despite the three different protections in place in the stomach, this bacterium attaches itself to the uppermost part of the stomach where it can stay away from the worst of the stomach acid. To make its home even cosier, it reduces the acidity around it (which means less stomach acid). This little bug can cause gastritis and ulcers [32]. Although for many people H. Pylori can be symptomless, for others, it can result in bloating, belching, nausea, vomiting and abdominal discomfort. In more severe cases, it can cause abdominal pain, decreased appetite, diarrhoea, and fatigue. It can also cause heartburn, low red blood cell count (anaemia), nausea and vomiting that may include vomiting blood, passing dark or tarry stools and peptic ulcers [33]. Vomiting blood or passing tarry stools should be referred to your doctor straight away. There is a lab test for H. Pylori (see Part III: Tests);

- You've something called a hiatal hernia. At the point where the oesophagus meets the stomach, it goes through an extensive muscle that covers the lower edge of your ribs, called the diaphragm. The diaphragm is there to help your lungs expand and contract properly to help you to breathe. If you've excess upward pressure in your stomach, this can cause part of the stomach to poke through the diaphragm like a little extra pouch. The causes of a hiatal hernia aren't well understood, but some candidates are pregnancy, obesity, coughing or even straining to pass a bowel movement [34]. It can sometimes cause symptoms of reflux and predisposes people to have issues with the inappropriate relaxation of the sphincter [35].

- Drinking water: some people believe that drinking water with your meal will dilute the pH of stomach acid and therefore result in upward pressure on the sphincter described above, as the stomach contents aren't broken down and stay in the stomach longer. However, a study carried out in 2008 showed that having a glass of water with your meal only affects the pH of the stomach for the first three minutes after drinking. After that, the pH level returns to its previous state [36]. However, the additional fluid will fill up the volume of the stomach and put further pressure on the sphincter muscle, so having a drink with your meal may still cause acid reflux.

While stomach acid production levels remain constant throughout life, the amount of pepsin that's produced declines with age [37], resulting in an overall reduction in the capability to break down food.

Your stomach can detect when food is sufficiently broken down to allow it to pass on to the next stage of digestion in the small intestine. If you don't break down your food enough, it will stay in the stomach longer, giving you symptoms of fullness, bloating, discomfort and sometimes lack of appetite (how can you eat if your body is still trying to digest the last thing you had?). Also, it will increase the upward pressure on the sphincter, as mentioned above. This force could cause stomach acid to escape into the oesophagus causing burning.

The Consequences of Long-Term Use of Proton Pump Inhibitors (PPIs)

In 1990, Omeprazole (Prilosec) was introduced to the US as the newest solution for excess stomach acid. In 2006, the consequences of long-term use of PPIs first started to appear. The Journal of the American Medical Association published a study associating higher risk of hip fractures in patients over the age of fifty with long-term use of PPI medicines. This is due to hypochlorhydria (low stomach acid) preventing sufficient absorption of calcium into the bone [38].

In May 2010 a study published in the journal Menopause found that post-menopausal women who take proton pump inhibitors may be 25% more likely to experience a bone fracture side effect [39].

In March 2011 a drug safety communication issued by the FDA in the US warned that 'prescription proton pump inhibitor (PPI) drugs might cause low serum magnesium levels (hypomagnesemia) if taken for prolonged periods of time.' Alongside that, the FDA issued a reminder that short-term use for fourteen days didn't cause problems [40].

In 2012 health officials in the UK warned that long-term use of proton pump inhibitors might result in an increased risk of bone fractures and cause dangerously low levels of magnesium in the body [41]. Very low magnesium levels have been associated with disturbances in nearly every organ system and potentially fatal complications (for example ventricular arrhythmia, coronary artery vasospasm and sudden death) [42].

In April 2016 the Journal of the American Medicine Association Neurology warned that PPIs might increase the risk of dementia in those aged over 75 by as much as 44% [43]. A further study indicated that patients taking proton pump inhibitor drugs might face an increased risk of chronic kidney disease and end-stage kidney failure [44].

Altogether this is a very bleak view of a family of very commonly prescribed drugs. If you stay on these medications for an extended period, you face the risks of bone loss and fractures, low magnesium levels, kidney disease and end-stage kidney failure and dementia.

36

Having said all this, please remember that short-term use (for a few weeks) doesn't cause problems. Medications are potent agents, and we should treat them with respect. If you are considering stopping a proton pump inhibitor, discuss this with your doctor. There are mixed views on whether a tapered dose avoids rebound hyperacidity or whether it doesn't make any difference [45] [46] [47] [48].

Sometimes PPIs are prescribed not for specific gastric conditions, such as reflux or gastric ulcers, but because several other medications are being taken together that could have an impact on the stomach (this is known as 'non-specific gastro-protection'). It's an 'off-license' use - it isn't the way PPIs are supposed to be used according to the drug manufacturers. Doctors use them as a precaution [49]. Given the severe side-effects noted for long-term use, this may warrant a conversation with your doctor. Always understand why you are taking any medication and for how long you should take it.

PPIs and Nutrient Deficiencies

Proton Pump Inhibitors obviously have an immediate effect on the acidity of the stomach. They could have a knock-on effect on the absorption of vitamins and minerals if you are elderly or you don't have a proper diet [50]. Proton pump inhibitors:

- Reduce magnesium absorption [51] [52] [53] – this is important for energy production, muscle relaxation, and heart health;

- Reduce calcium absorption [54]– this is important for bone strength;

- Reduce production of vitamin B12 [55] – this is important for energy production;

- Reduce iron [56]– this is important for oxygen delivery to tissues;

- Reduce vitamin C – vitamin C becomes less stable in less acidic environments [57]. Vitamin C is a crucial antioxidant which protects the body from harmful free radicals;

- Reduce zinc – increased pH inhibits break down of proteins in the stomach and zinc becomes 'less available' to the body [58]. Zinc is essential for a robust immune system, skin health, and the capability to make new proteins and DNA;

- Loosens 'tight junctions' in the gut [59]. Gaps then allow undigested particles of food to enter the body where they come under scrutiny from the immune system (IgG) and can potentially lead to new food sensitivities, along with all the symptoms previously mentioned.

The seriousness of these effects does depend on your state of health. For example, if your zinc intake from food is low then a further decrease due to the action of PPIs will be more significant, whereas if your diet is rich in zinc a reduction may not make a noticeable difference.

There is also a potential increase in small intestinal bacterial overgrowth (known as SIBO) [60] [61]. SIBO is covered in more detail under the FODMAPS section. SIBO happens when there are excessive bacteria in the small intestine and, consequently, cause many people to suffer from chronic diarrhoea and be unable to absorb nutrients from their food. SIBO further reduces vitamin B12.

The Science behind Food Intolerances – Beyond the Stomach

Anytime we eat food our body releases a whole cascade of enzymes to break it down from large molecules to small molecules. Different enzymes break down the various food groups - fats, carbohydrates (sugars) and proteins. This breakdown starts in the mouth with amylase in saliva, which begins to break down carbohydrates. Chew a piece of bread for longer than you would usually and you'll notice it starts to taste sweet – this is because amylase has begun to break down the carbohydrate into sugars.

Many enzymes are produced in the pancreas and then squirted into the small intestine to work on food breakdown. These are lipase (which works with bile from the liver to break down fats), protease (to break down proteins) and more amylase (to break down carbohydrates). Any of these enzymes could be deficient.

Lack of lipase results in a lack of needed fats and inability to absorb fat-soluble vitamins A, D, E, and K. Obvious symptoms are diarrhoea and fatty stools that float on the surface of the water in the toilet bowl.

Lack of protease results in the inability to break down proteins. It makes it a lot harder to keep the intestine free of parasites. It's more likely that you may suffer from allergies, intolerances and sensitivities and it increases the risk of intestinal infections.

Lack of amylase results in diarrhoea due to body's attempts to get rid of undigested starch in the colon [62].

People with cystic fibrosis or pancreatic cancer have severe issues with pancreatic enzyme *deficiency* and will take supplemental enzymes as part of their medication regime [63], but enzyme *insufficiency* is prevalent in the general population. Eating foods which contain enzymes (see Part IV: Solutions), eating foods that prompt the pancreas to produce more enzymes, or taking enzyme supplements will help. Work with a practitioner to find the best choice for you.

Pancreatic enzymes don't work very well if you take antacids such as Gaviscon, Tums or Rennies. These medicines reduce acidity. Not only are you affecting what happens in your stomach (less breakdown) but you are also changing what happens in the next stage after that.

Intestinal Permeability, or 'Leaky Gut'

Hippocrates, the father of modern medicine, said: "All disease begins in the gut," and so it does. When things go wrong in the gut, all sorts of allergies, intolerances, sensitivities and diseases are possible. Even in the 1980s researchers investigated the physiology of the intestines (how they work) and used the phrase 'intestinal permeability' [64] [65].

When food reaches your intestines, it's in a liquid state. On exiting the stomach, the action of the various enzymes should be to break down the remaining molecules until each one is tiny.

When they're broken down in that way, they can diffuse (spread) through the cell membranes as expected to give you all their nourishment without causing any problems. Nothing big can get through the cell membranes. However, the space between the cells is another matter.

The cells are joined together by special glue-like bonds. Some substances will dissolve the 'glue,' and more substantial molecules will be able to get through this gap into the inside of the body. It sets in motion the immune IgG-mediated antibody response, which will determine whether that substance is tolerated or becomes a food sensitivity.

You already know how food sensitivities can result in just about any condition, affecting just about any part of the body. The stage is set not just for sensitivities but also a range of autoimmune diseases and cancer [66] [67].

The common term for intestinal permeability is leaky gut, and it can be caused by anything that enables larger, undigested particles of food to traverse the small intestine, break the bonds between cells and exit where they shouldn't, into the body. These include:

Gliadin (a part of gluten) [68]; milk proteins [69]; medications: non-steroidal anti-inflammatory drugs such as ibuprofen (advil and motrin in the US) and indomethacin (indocin in the US)), and aspirin [70] [71]; smoking [72]; alcohol [73]; and food additives [74].

Part II: The Foods

Gluten (Gluten is a Top 14 Allergen)

Gluten is one of the Top 14 Allergens. Gluten is a protein that we associate mostly with wheat, but it's also in spelt, barley and rye. Anyone who has issues with gluten may also need to avoid those other grains; you can check this with a food intolerance test or by excluding gluten from your diet. If your symptoms don't improve after removing it, you may need to look for other gluten-containing culprits.

Gluten is biochemically similar to proteins in other grains, such as oats and corn. There is more information about these later.

Gluten and Coeliac Disease

I've included Coeliac Disease to dispel a few myths, as many people think of it as a form of severe allergy and worry that if their gluten intolerance becomes very severe, it may become Coeliac disease. Coeliac (pronounced 'see-lee-ack') disease isn't an allergy or a food intolerance but an autoimmune disease. 'Autoimmune' means the body attacks itself.

Coeliac disease only occurs when there is the 'perfect storm' of specific genetic influences, specific environmental impacts (this term is used in its broadest sense of how a person lives their life as well as where they live it) and certain foods.

People aren't born with Coeliac disease, but they may have genes which predispose them to Coeliac disease at some time in their lives - having the gene *might* mean you develop Coeliac disease but it doesn't mean you'll acquire it. The most common genes are called HLA-DQ2.5, HLA-DQ8 and finally HLA-DQ2.8.

About 40% of the population have these genes. You could inherit just one copy of one of these genes, meaning a lower risk of progressing to the disease, or two copies, one from each parent, in which case there is a higher risk of progressing to the disease. Only 1% of the population in total will go on to develop Coeliac disease [75].

The HLA genes cause the immune cells in the lining of the small intestine to recognise gluten as an invader and create an inflammatory response, which damages the gut lining. Over time, this results in stunted growth of the 'carpet' that lines the small intestine (called 'villi' – see below for the science).

Stunted growth of the villi makes it more difficult to absorb nutrients from food, and the person becomes malnourished and very sick. They can sometimes (but not always) lose a lot of weight. As coeliac disease is a 'systemic' (whole body) disease, there could also be symptoms elsewhere in the body.

Environmental influences that can make you more disposed to being Coeliac are:

- Having a close family member who is also Coeliac;

- Having other autoimmune diseases, such as type 1 diabetes, Downs, Turner or Williams syndromes, or thyroid disease [75]. Between 4% and 9% of people with type 1 diabetes also have diagnosed Coeliac disease, compared with 1% in the general population without type 1 diabetes (there is no increased risk for type 2 diabetics as type 2 diabetes isn't an auto-immune disease). Between 1% and 4% of people with thyroid disease (Hashimoto's or Graves') is Coeliac, compared with one percent in the general population without thyroid disease.

A further factor in the development of Coeliac disease is, of course, food. The situation would be more straightforward if wheat were the only grain containing gluten, but it isn't. Coeliacs also must avoid spelt, barley and rye grains. Furthermore, gluten is the substance that makes bread stretchy and light. Many processed foods use this same quality. Gluten is in everything from bread to gravy granules, from pasta to pizza, and anything containing batter or breadcrumbs. It's also in some ready-made sauces.

For a very detailed description of what is gluten-free, what to check and what to avoid, see A Guide to Eating Gluten-Free in Part V: Helpful Resources.

It's worth pointing out that there are some foods that do contain gluten included in the gluten-free column of the guide, such as barley, malt vinegar and Worcestershire sauce. This is because, although they do contain a trace amount of gluten, this amount in relation to the quantity likely to be eaten at any one time is below the threshold of tolerance for most Coeliacs and therefore is permissible.

Foods such as suet, on the other hand, *aren't* gluten free in the guide, even though they're just fat and shouldn't contain gluten at all. There could be a cross-contamination risk that can't be quantified. It's always useful to check the label if you aren't sure.

Modern strains of wheat have proteins that are more likely to result in an allergic response than older varieties [76].

The Science Behind Coeliac Disease

The role of your small intestine is to break down food chemically into tiny particles that can then be absorbed and used for energy throughout your body – food breakdown gives you the raw materials. If you were to look at the inside surface of the small intestine under a microscope, you would see a row of densely packed fronds that look like a shag-pile carpet. These are called villi. On the top of these, there is another shag-pile carpet called microvilli. The point of all this carpeting is to increase the surface area in your gut massively so that it meets more food particles and can absorb more of them.

In Coeliac disease, gluten scrubs away at your shag-pile carpet, literally rubbing it away until there is none left. Not only does this reduce the surface area available for absorption of nutrients, but it also means you can't absorb nutrients because the whole mechanism with which to do so is now missing.

If left untreated it can have severe consequences; it's a life-long condition that requires constant vigilance. The only treatment is to avoid all gluten in wheat and other gluten-containing grains and to be rigorous in preventing contamination in the same kitchen, using the same utensils and chopping boards, whether in the home or commercial kitchens if you are eating out. The slightest bit of gluten does make a difference –

Coeliacs should avoid any kitchen surface previously used for gluten – even the toaster!

Symptoms of Coeliac Disease

The symptoms of Coeliac disease could include any of the following:
Anaemia, bloating, constipation, diarrhoea, flatulence, hair loss, headache, mouth ulcers, nausea, tiredness, sudden weight loss, and osteoporosis.

More than a Gluten Free Diet

There are some situations where a gluten-free diet alone doesn't seem to resolve the symptoms. In these cases, there could also be small intestine bacterial overgrowth (SIBO) or lactose intolerance as secondary features (see lactose intolerance section later). A small study of twelve patients carried out in a gastroenterology clinic over a three-year period showed that resolution of these issues resulted in complete success when paired with a gluten-free diet [77].

Avenin and Coeliac Disease

Oats contain a protein called avenin, which has a very similar biochemical structure to gluten. You'll find 'gluten-free oats' in the supermarkets. It means these oats grew in an area where there are no gluten-containing crops in nearby fields, and the factories that processed the oats don't process gluten. It seems to be sufficient for most people who are on a gluten-free diet [78] [79] and may also be beneficial for Coeliacs. However, the introduction of oats should be managed under medical supervision as not all Coeliacs can tolerate oats [80] [81].

Potential Nutrient Deficiencies for Coeliacs

The minerals iron and calcium, and the vitamins folate, vitamin B12, and all the fat-soluble vitamins (A, D, E, and K) can't be absorbed when the villi and microvilli (the 'shag pile carpet') are worn away. Deficiencies can lead to diseases such as osteoporosis, lymphoma and small bowel cancer. Once a Coeliac has completely removed gluten from his diet the 'carpet' regenerates, and he can absorb these vitamins and minerals once more. The additional disease risks of osteoporosis, lymphoma and small bowel cancer also reduce [82].

Non-Coeliac Gluten Sensitivity

Non-Coeliac-Gluten-Sensitivity is also on the increase [83]. It's the term that doctors give gluten sensitivity to distinguish it from either Coeliac disease or wheat allergy. Symptoms appear soon after eating gluten and have a 'classic' irritable bowel presentation of abdominal pain, bloating, diarrhoea, or constipation, and 'foggy head.' There can also be a headache, fatigue, joint and muscle pain, leg or arm numbness, dermatitis (eczema or skin rash), depression and anaemia.

The most common symptoms in children are abdominal pain, chronic diarrhoea and tiredness [84] [85]. Gluten sensitivity doesn't cause any damage to the intestinal 'carpet' in the way that Coeliac disease does.

Wheat Production in 2017

Here is the output from the most significant producers of wheat in 2017:

- European Union - 150.754 million tons;

- China - 131 million tons;

- India - 96 million tons;

- Russia - 69 million tons.

The US produced 49.642 million tons [86]. The total world output of wheat for 2017/18 is forecast at 754.8 million tons. This output is 1% lower than 2016. Wheat utilisation in 2017/18 is forecast at 740 million tonnes. Food consumption of wheat is set to expand by 1.1%, to an all-time high of 504 million tonnes [87]. Wheat is becoming a bigger part of our diet.

How often do we hear the older generation say: "things aren't what they used to be…"? In the case of wheat, they're right. Gluten intolerance was unheard of in previous generations. So, what has changed? Wheat processing changed massively in the 19th century to remove the wheat germ and wheat bran. Unfortunately, that's where the grain stores most of the nutrients. The inferior product that was left causes rapid spikes in blood sugar without the starchy carbohydrates from fibre to slow it down.

Varieties of Wheat

Botanists have identified over 30,000 different types of wheat. These are assigned to different classifications depending on the season in which they grow and their nutrient composition: hard red winter, hard red spring, soft red winter, durum, hard white and soft white. The varieties of wheat are classified according to the protein-to-starch ratio in the endosperm (the starchy middle of the seed). Hard wheats contain more protein and less starch [88]. Even though there is so much choice, 90% of the wheat grown throughout the world comes from just a few varieties [89].

Wheat Nutrient Profile since 1843

Fortunately, we do have records of wheat growth characteristics going back to 1843, when the Broadwalk Experiment was established in the Rothamsted Agricultural Research station. This was an exercise in measuring the growing conditions of wheat (and the nutrient values of the wheat that was produced). It was in existence for over a hundred years – in fact, it's still in existence today [90]. We can see from their records that the amount of zinc, copper, iron, and magnesium was consistent from the time of the establishment until the 1960s.

The 1960s was when growers introduced semi-dwarf, high-yielding varieties of wheat. Wheat has been selectively bred to enhance its elastic properties and change the gluten structure since then. Intense cross-breeding programs have turned the crop into something neither physically nor genetically like its old self.

Old wheat varieties grew more than four feet tall. Modern wheat (found in 99 percent of the world's wheat fields) is now called 'dwarf wheat,' standing just two feet in height with an abnormally large seed head balanced atop its stocky stem, to make it easier for machines to harvest [91]. Trends show decreasing nutrient concentrations in the wheat: iron and zinc levels are particularly affected [92] [93]. The farmers are producing more grain with less nutrient value.

"The Dose Makes the Poison"

As if there weren't enough problems with wheat already, fungicides, pesticides and herbicides are sprayed onto crops. The seeds are sprayed with fungicides and pesticides even before planting [94]. In 2012, there were nineteen different treatment options for seeds (various fungicides and pesticides) and thirty-six different ingredients that could be used beyond the seed stage to control multiple plant diseases that may infect wheat [95].

The herbicide glyphosate, otherwise known as 'Roundup,' is sprayed just before harvest to dry the grain and speed up the time to reach harvest by as much as two weeks. This practice began in Scotland in the 1980s when the crops were too wet to harvest. Glyphosate is a desiccant for this purpose. This practice is commonplace across the US now.

The global conglomerate, Monsanto, produces Glyphosate. Glyphosate is the subject of a great deal of controversy, with a research paper by French molecular biologist Gilles-Éric Séralini claiming proven toxicity published and then retracted after Monsanto officials were appointed to the board of the journal that published the paper [96] [97].

There followed a series of accusations, counter-accusations, lawsuits and publications by both the original author and various experts in support or denial of his case [98]. Glyphosate has been implicated in cancer as well as endocrine disruption affecting male and female fertility [99] [100] [101] [102] [103].

It has also been implicated in issues with the health of mitochondria (involved in energy creation), skin membranes [104], bowel motility [105] and more. Subsequent studies concerning the safety of glyphosate are continuing to generate the same level of disagreement and debate.

Glyphosate was initially considered safe for humans (and many research studies commissioned by its creators, Monsanto, and associated interests support this). It was due to the minimal residues remaining in food. The definition of a 'safe dose' uses the principle of using high-dose testing to predict low-dose results, called "The dose makes the poison." This principle has been in place since the 1600s and has been used for safety testing of any chemical since then, from pesticides to plastics.

Endocrinologists (doctors who specialise in hormones), don't support this high-dose testing principle. These people understand how tiny amounts of hormones (or substances that behave like hormones) can make a huge difference to human function. Recently, health officials have recognised glyphosate as an endocrine disruptor. High-dose testing doesn't predict low-dose results. According to the endocrinologists, the smaller the dose, the more potent it could be [106].

In 2015 the World Health Organisation said glyphosate was a *probable* carcinogen (it could cause cancer), but then subsequently retracted the statement following fierce criticism about its research methods. California listed it as a carcinogen in 2017 [107] [108]. Whether it is or it isn't, this has huge implications for health, industry and jobs worldwide. No doubt this debate will continue for many years to come.

It's still possible to buy old varieties of wheat like emmer, einkorn and Kamut, but these are specialities rather than the norm. These grains cause fewer allergic and sensitivity reactions [109].

Gluten affects IBS symptoms [110]. A gluten-free diet may mean this condition is reversible [111].

Bread-Making
The process of bread-making has also substantially changed: wheat grains used to be sprouted to activate the health-giving nutrients. (See solutions for how to sprout). They were fermented to break down proteins. The yeast was slow-rise, which meant it worked in the bread for longer. Yeast multiplies using the carbohydrate as food but breaks down gluten in the process (a process we see now only in traditional sourdough). It needs time to break down the gluten [112] [113] [114].

'Gluten-Free' on Food Labels
In January 2009, European Commission (EC) Regulation No 47 41/2009 concerning the composition and labelling of foodstuffs suitable for people intolerant to gluten became law. The regulation defined:

- 'Very low gluten' as gluten content not exceeding 100 mg/kg. (This is 100 parts per million);

- 'Gluten-free' as gluten content not exceeding 20 mg/kg (This is 20 parts per million).

A study has shown that for Coeliacs a daily gluten intake of fewer than 10 mg per day is unlikely to cause significant damage to the intestinal villi (the 'shag pile carpet') [115].

I wonder what happens in the 'grey zone' in between 10 parts per million and 20 parts per million? While 'gluten-free' goods made from wheat, spelt, barley or rye (these are the grains that contain gluten) are acceptable for anyone with gluten sensitivity, the amount of gluten remaining in these grains may still be above the threshold for Coeliacs, and it's possible they may experience symptoms.

Most gluten-free goods use combinations of grains (like rice and potato) that are gluten-free in the first place, so this isn't an issue.

Care also needs to be taken with sourdough bread. Traditional sourdough manufacture uses a sourdough starter with bacteria. The bacteria ferment over seven days and produce gas, which makes the dough rise. The fermentation also causes the gluten protein to be broken down, thus making it suitable for people who are gluten-intolerant but not for Coeliacs. Sourdough bread made in this way doesn't use yeast.

The sourdough bread available in supermarkets is made quickly with yeast. It may still have the tangy taste of sourdough, but it won't contain the bacteria and therefore will still contain the gluten. Avoid bread that says 'sourdough style' if you've any issues with gluten.

Gluten-Containing Foods and Products

Top Tips: If you are sensitive to gluten, look out for these foods:

> Barley (including products that contain malted barley such as malted drinks, beers, ales, lagers, and stouts). Bulgur wheat, couscous, durum wheat, einkorn, emmer (also known as faro),

Khorasan wheat (commercially known as kamut®), pearl barley, rye, semolina, spelt, triticale, and wheat [116].

Top Tips: these products may contain gluten:
Baking powder, batter, breadcrumbs, cakes, flour, meat products, oven foods like chips (potato fries), pasta, pastry, sauces, and soups.

Gluten Free Foods

The market for gluten-free foodstuffs is booming. According to Euromonitor, the consumer data group, global sales of gluten-free food were $1.7bn in 2011 and had risen to $3.5bn in 2016. Euromonitor estimated that figure could reach $4.7bn by 2020.

There are many reasons for this trend. Part of it is due to Coeliacs and other people who *must* have gluten-free foods to avoid serious health issues, including those with other autoimmune diseases [117]. Part of it is due to a growing understanding of food sensitivities. Some people also believe that eating gluten-free is a healthier diet.

Should everyone be gluten-free? Not according to a small study published in the British Journal of Nutrition, which found that in a group of healthy adults given a gluten-free diet, populations of healthy gut bacteria decreased [118].

'Healthy adults' meant no history of digestive pathology or signs of malnutrition. None of the volunteers had been treated with antibiotics for at least two months before the faecal sampling. I believe that the definition of 'healthy' should be a lot broader than just 'not having digestive pathology'. Similarly, I wonder what constituted the 'healthy diet' (information not supplied in the study) if the removal of gluten could make such a difference.

Our Western diet relies heavily on gluten and cereals, and if we had the right balance, including a rainbow of colours in our daily fruits and vegetables, many of our modern illnesses would be rare [119] [120] [121]. Food manufacturers are working very, very hard to produce gluten-free bread that's light and fluffy and as palatable as wheat bread (because that's what consumers want), but they also need to work on

51

the nutrition and what it does inside our bodies, for the benefit of everyone who eats it.

Food manufacturing with a focus on nutrition is a new trend though. Read the label on a gluten-free loaf, and you'll see it contains myriad ingredients, many of which are names you probably don't recognise. It isn't as simple as just replacing one flour for another. Other grains don't have the stretchiness of gluten, but that's what we demand. How much the findings of this study were down to the gluten and how much down to other substances in the gluten-free substitutes, we don't know.

Gluten, Casein, and ASD (Autistic Spectrum Disorder)

ASD is a group of developmental disabilities that includes autism and Asperger's syndrome. Individuals with ASD may have problems with verbal and non-verbal communications, difficulties with social interaction and tend towards repetitive behaviours or narrow, obsessive interests. While the full development of the condition isn't known, there are many possible causes. One persistent theory called the 'Opioid-Excess theory' involves a combination of insufficient enzymatic activity (breaking things down), increased intestinal permeability (leaky gut) and, consequently, the absorption of proteins from gluten and casein [122].

Research has reported abnormal levels of gluten and casein peptides (fragments of proteins) in the urine and cerebrospinal fluid (the fluid that's found in the brain and spinal chord) of people with autism [123]. There are reports that a gluten-free and casein-free (GFCF) diet may help children with these conditions communicate more efficiently and improve overall well-being [110] [124].

Wheat Allergy

The Nutritional Profile of Wheat

Wheat is an essential source of manganese, tryptophan and magnesium. The benefits of all vitamins, minerals and other nutrients are listed in Part V: Helpful Resources.

Wheat Allergy Proteins and Symptoms

Wheat Allergy is an IgE-mediated reaction to one of the proteins in wheat. It could be a reaction to gluten, but it could be a reaction to albumin, globulin, gliadin (one of the two components of gluten) or glutenin (the other part of gluten). This immune response can affect the respiratory system.

Known since the Roman Empire, baker's asthma and rhinitis are well-characterised allergic reactions to inhaling wheat flours, affecting up to 10%-15% of bakers, millers, and pastry factory workers [125].

Most wheat-allergic children suffer from moderate-to-severe atopic dermatitis (a condition that makes your skin red and itchy), and they may experience urticaria (a skin rash with red, raised and itchy bumps), facial swelling, nausea, bronchial obstruction and abdominal pain or, in severe cases, anaphylaxis. They often outgrow it by school age, similar to the way milk or egg allergies can disappear by this time [126].

This allergy requires avoidance of any food containing wheat. Non-food items with wheat-based ingredients such as Play-Doh, cosmetics or bath products can also cause an allergic reaction [4].

Cross-Reactivity – Wheat and Exercise

The most common adult presentation of this allergy is an exercise-induced allergy. Gastrointestinal symptoms could be mild and difficult to recognise; the most common are diarrhoea and bloating. Eating wheat without exercise doesn't cause a problem, and exercise without eating wheat doesn't create a problem, but there is a problem when the two occur together [127].

Filaggrin Gene Mutation

Genes act as instructions to make proteins. They're 'recipes'. Every person has two copies of each gene, one inherited from each parent. Most genes are the same in all people, but less than 1% of our genes are slightly different between people. These differences are called 'mutations', and they contribute to each person's unique physical features [128].

One gene associated with the skin is called Filaggrin. According to the US National Library of Medicine:

> *"Filaggrin plays an important role in the skin's barrier function. It brings together structural proteins in the outermost skin cells to form tight bundles, flattening and strengthening the cells to create a strong barrier."*

It also helps maintain hydration of the skin and the correct acidity (pH) of the skin, which is another important aspect of the skin barrier [129] [130].

People with this gene mutation are often susceptible to eczema. A total of 3,471 adults completed a questionnaire about food allergies and had a health examination. The answers to the questionnaire revealed a connection between mutations in the filaggrin gene and allergies to egg, fish, milk, wheat, and sensitivity to alcohol. Subsequent IgE antibody tests confirmed the cross-relationship with milk and the sensitivity to alcohol [131].

Avocado

Avocados are a fantastic addition to your diet – not only are they full of nutrients, but the healthy fat content enables you to absorb more nutrients, such as vitamin A [132] and carotenoids [133] from other foods you eat alongside them. You'll find the highest phytonutrient concentration in the darker green flesh next to the skin, so make sure you leave none of that behind when you eat it.

The Health Benefits of Avocado

Avocados are known to support cardiovascular health, blood sugar control, insulin regulation, eyesight, satiety (feeling full) and weight management [134] [135], as well as lowering inflammation [136].

The Nutritional Profile of Avocado

They contain vitamins B5, B6, C, E, and K, copper, folate, fibre, potassium and lutein [137].

Intolerance to Avocado

If you have issues with avocado, they could be due to sorbitol, salicylates, or amines. These are natural compounds in the avocado that are well tolerated by most people.

For more information on amines, see the Histamine section. For more information on salicylates – see the Salicylates section. Sorbitol is a sugar alcohol, known as a polyol. For more information on the actions of polyols, see the FODMAPS section.

The symptoms of intolerance to avocado could be any of the following:

> Abdominal pain, bloating, changes in bowel movements, excessive flatulence.

Top Tips: if you are sensitive to avocados:

- Check the ingredients in vegan and paleo recipes, as they may use avocado to add creaminess instead of using dairy products;

- Avocado is a substitute for butter or other fats in some recipes;

- In baked goods, avocado adds a fluffy texture; it's even used in some chocolate chip cookie and brownie recipes, and, my personal favourite, chocolate ice cream! [138].

Beef

The French used to call the British "Les Rosbifs," due to the amount of beef we ate. According to Mintel, beef isn't favoured as much these days, with over a quarter (28%) of meat-eating Brits reducing or limiting their meat consumption in the six months to August 2017. A further one in seven (14%) adults say they're considering reducing their consumption of meat or poultry in the future [139].

The Health Benefits of Beef

Animal protein is very high in the nine essential amino acids we need. It makes beef one of the most 'complete' sources of protein.

The Nutritional Profile of Beef

Beef is rich in vitamins B2, B3, B6, B5, B12, omega-3 fats, zinc, selenium, iron, potassium, phosphorous and choline [140].

Potential Problems with Beef

Why does beef cause a problem? Issues can extend from full-blown allergy (although this is currently very rare in the UK) to food sensitivity (much more common). A tick bite in humans may consequently cause the allergy [141]. It's very unusual in that this immune IgE-mediated allergy reaction isn't to a protein but to a carbohydrate called 'alpha-gal,' found in beef and other meats such as pork and lamb.

Poultry such as chicken or turkey doesn't have this carbohydrate [142]. It can result in anaphylactic shock, which leads to the airways closing, and therefore it can be life-threatening. It can follow the usual pattern for severe allergies - occurring immediately after eating the food - or it can happen in a novel form with delayed allergic responses up to three hours later.

The 'alpha-gal' phenomenon is common in the southern, central, and eastern US. In 2006, the first instance was recorded in Australia [143], and it has since appeared in countries of Asia and Europe, including the UK. Early indications are that drinking alcohol at the same time as eating red meat increases the probability of a reaction [142]. It could be because alcohol opens the tight junctions between cells in the gut.

Beef is a very rich source of protein and, as we know, proteins are the things that can be identified as foreign invaders when fragments get in the wrong places in the body. There can be a sensitivity reaction producing any of the following symptoms:

> Abdominal pain, bloating, diarrhoea, excessive gas, fatigue, hives, nausea, runny nose, sneezing, stomach cramps or vomiting.

Another issue with beef relates to cooking temperatures. When you cook meats at high temperatures, the heat produces a set of chemicals called heterocyclic amines (HCAs). Scientists measured more than seventeen different types of HCAs in meat cooked at high temperatures. Stewing, barbecuing and frying appear to produce the most HCAs. Gravies made from meat juices also have a high amine content (see separate section on amines). These chemicals need to be broken down by efficient liver detoxification.

Top Tip: if you are sensitive to beef - make sure you are eating broccoli and other cruciferous vegetables (cauliflower, brussels sprouts, kale, bok choy and rocket, known as arugula in the US) every week to assist liver detoxification.

Celery (This is a Top 14 Allergen)

The Health Benefits of Celery

Celery is anti-inflammatory, especially in the digestive tract. Celery contains high levels of anti-oxidants, which are substances that repair the 'wear and tear' damage caused in our bodies daily - some of these aren't affected by cooking so you can still get the benefits.

The Nutritional Profile of Celery

Celery has excellent levels of copper, calcium, folate, magnesium molybdenum, phosphorous, potassium, fibre, manganese and vitamins A, B5, B6, B12 and K.

Celery Allergy

Celery is a pervasive allergen in France, Germany, and Switzerland although less so in the UK. However, it can be severe. Contact with the stalk, leaves, seeds, root or oil of the plant can all cause the allergy.

A local allergic reaction will affect just your skin, mouth and throat, but a severe allergic response could release large amounts of histamine and other chemicals and even result in anaphylaxis. There is a link between allergy to pollen and celery (see Oral Allergy Syndrome later) [144].

Celery allergy causes rashes, leading to hives, asthma, contact dermatitis, facial swelling and possibly anaphylaxis. It can also increase photosensitivity in people who work with celery in food shops or who pick celery. The celery releases toxic chemicals that protect it from predators. It can result in skin blistering after just a little sun exposure. Various forms of fungus can increase celery's photosensitising capability massively. This feature seems to be at its height before the plant is visibly diseased, so only ever use celery in perfect condition. This reaction is caused by touching the plant, not by eating it.

A study comparing prepared solutions of healthy and diseased celery placed in contact with the forearm for just one minute produced some very startling results: The fresh celery produced no reaction, but the infected celery caused severe reddening of the skin within two days and skin blistering after a week. It took six weeks for the blistering to heal, but pigmentation was still visible after three months [145].

Distribution and storage may play a part in the disease process. One of these studies states the time between harvest and consumption was only four days, so if you are considering a bite for lunch and see that tired, floppy celery lurking at the bottom of your fridge that has been there for days – just put it straight in the bin! [146]

Top Tips: if you are sensitive to celery, look out for these foods -
The celery plant, celeriac and celery salt. You also need to check labels for processed meat products as they may contain celery as seasoning.

Top Tips: these products may contain celery -
Soups, spice mixes, and salad dressings [147].

Heating doesn't destroy celery allergens. If you have a celery allergy, you should avoid it whether it's cooked or raw.

Citrus

Citrus fruits are probably best known for their valuable vitamin C and the role this played in correcting the disease called scurvy. Scurvy was described as long ago as the ancient Egyptians, and then subsequently by the Greeks and Romans. It continued to plague both sailors and populations without adequate access to fruit and vegetables.

58

Fortunately, it's rare these days, but it's characterised by weakness, feeling sad and irritable all the time, severe joint or leg pain, swollen and bleeding gums, skin that bruises easily and red or blue spots on the shins. Severe vitamin C deficiency can occur within only three months if people don't eat fruit and vegetables [148].

The Health Benefits of Citrus

Citrus is a good source of soluble and insoluble fibre, keeping you 'regular' and also feeding your gut bacteria at the same time. It contains flavonoids which are good for heart health (but don't eat grapefruit if you take statins. It interferes with the way the drug works).

Although citrus can taste sweet, it won't spike your blood sugar – the glucose is steadily released so that you can maintain your energy without a 'sugar crash' later (please note, this applies to the whole fruit and not concentrated fruit juices. Without the entire fruit fibre, juice can be broken down rapidly, allowing a flood of glucose into your system. That's just from the sugar in the fruit. On top of that, consider up to sixteen teaspoons of added sugar that make that drink so temptingly sweet, and you have the perfect recipe for a severe blood sugar spike, followed by a blood sugar crash: hunger, possibly moodiness, fatigue, or a headache).

Citrus may reduce the duration of colds by supporting your immune system. There is also a significant benefit in eating citrus with other foods, such as leafy greens, fish, poultry and meat. These foods contain iron, which is sometimes hard for your body to absorb. The vitamin C increases the rate of iron absorption from the same amount of food. It also keeps you hydrated, due to its high-water content.

The Nutritional Profile of Citrus

People think of citrus as an excellent source of vitamin C. However, like most other whole foods, citrus fruits also contain an impressive list of other essential nutrients:

> Vitamins A, B2, B3, B5, B6, and C. Copper, calcium, folate, magnesium, potassium, thiamin, phosphorus and a variety of phytochemicals (biologically active compounds).

Citrus Allergy

Citrus allergy isn't very common, but there can be cross-reactivity to grass pollen (see Oral Allergy Syndrome).

Oils in citrus peel from lemons, limes and oranges contain chemicals called furocoumarins. If exposure to sunlight follows contact with citrus, this can result in phototoxicity reactions causing a red, itchy skin rash in sensitive people [149].

Citric acid in its natural form from fruit doesn't cause allergies.

Corn

Are you confused by the difference between maize and corn? The US grows over 90 million acres of corn each year, but 99% of that isn't for human consumption. The kind that we eat is known as sweetcorn (Zea mays convar. saccharate convar. rugosa). It's harvested in the summer when the kernels still taste sweet (hence the name).

The rest of the corn is a different variety known as field corn (Zea mays indentata). It grows taller than sweetcorn and has thicker leaves, and it isn't sweet! It's left in the fields for the kernels to dry out, mostly because that makes it easier to process. Although some of it makes corn meal, corn chips and corn syrup, most of it becomes animal feed [150].

The Health Benefits of Corn

Sweetcorn is famous for the fact that the kernels don't seem to be very digestible. Congratulations for noticing one of the benefits of sweetcorn – it's high in insoluble fibre. It's good to help food transit time through your bowel, but there is soluble fibre there as well, together with a range of vitamins and other nutrients [151].

Have you ever given any thought to the threads called 'corn silks' covering the corn inside the cob, or do you throw them away? These long, silky fibres that run along the length of the cobs are very health-giving. You can make a tea with them. Corn silk can help reduce bladder infections and inflammation of the urinary system and prostate, kidney stones and bedwetting.

How does it work? Corn silk contains proteins, carbohydrates, vitamins, minerals and fibre. It also includes chemicals that seem to work like diuretics, enabling the body to lose excess water, and it may help reduce inflammation [152].

The Nutritional Profile of Corn
Corn is rich in Vitamin B3, B5, B6, manganese and phosphorous.

Corn Allergy
Corn allergy is unusual, and reactions tend to be mild.

Corn Intolerance
The inability to fully digest the protein in corn, called zein, causes corn intolerance. It's a substantial protein and has a similar structure to gluten. It can lead to leaky gut. Due to the gluten-like structure, it may be better to avoid it if you are Coeliac.

Crustaceans (These are Top 14 Allergens)

A few standard terms need some definition here: people use the words 'shellfish' and 'seafood' interchangeably, but seafood includes fish whereas shellfish doesn't. Shellfish does include both crustaceans and molluscs. Crustaceans number 44,000 species of animal that live in water and have a hard outer shell.

They're amongst the most common causes of food allergies and are the third most important cause of food-induced anaphylaxis. Allergies towards crustaceans last a lifetime and commonly appear at a later stage of life [153].

Symptoms occur on eating the food, touching it or inhaling the steam from cooking it. Boiling shrimp can increase the allergenic reaction due to a chemical process called the 'Maillard reaction.' This allergy is a major problem in countries that have a significant shellfish processing industry or where shellfish is a popular food. There are several potential protein allergens, but the most common one is called tropomyosin.

The Nutritional Profile of Crustaceans

Crustaceans are high in choline, copper, iodine, selenium, vitamins A, B3, B5, B6, B12 and E, phosphorous, zinc and omega-3 fats.

Crustacean Cross-Reactivity

There can be cross-reactivity to other foods within the crustacean family and to house dust mites, midges, moths and cockroaches as these have similar proteins to tropomyosin. There can also be cross-reactions to molluscs (which are themselves another top 14 allergen) and cod worm.

Top Tips: if you are sensitive to crustaceans, look out for these foods - Crab, crayfish, langoustine, lobster, shrimps, scampi and prawns.

Top Tips: shrimp paste may contain crustacean - Asian cooking uses this paste widely.

Shellfish Poisoning

Shellfish poisoning can produce the same sort of symptoms as an allergy, depending on the amount of shellfish eaten and the level of toxins it may have. There are five different types of shellfish poisoning [154], as well as adverse reactions to bacterial or viral contamination from Clostridium botulinum, staphylococcal enterotoxin or Norovirus (also called the Winter Vomiting Bug).

Shellfish poisoning can produce a wide variety of symptoms depending on the toxin concerned, including nausea, vomiting, diarrhoea, dizziness, numbness, tingling or burning of lips, tongue and throat, and even temporary paralysis.

Symptoms can occur between half an hour to three hours after eating [155]. Fortunately, the effects don't reoccur if you eat the same food again but many people who have had a severe bout of food poisoning may develop such a strong aversion to the food that they'll never eat it again.

Eggs (These are Top 14 Allergens)

It takes a hen between 24 to 26 hours to produce an egg. Hens produce bigger eggs as they grow older. Eggs age more in one day at room temperature than they do in one week in the refrigerator [156], so store them appropriately.

The Health Benefits of Eggs

Eggs are an excellent source of high-quality protein. They're regarded as a 'complete' source of protein as they contain all nine essential amino acids - the ones we can't make in our bodies and must obtain from our diet.

The Nutritional Profile of Eggs

Eggs are an excellent source of vitamins A, B2, B5, B12, D, E and K, calcium, choline, folic acid, iodine, iron, lutein, zeaxanthin, phosphorous, selenium and zinc.

Eggs and Cholesterol

Eggs are high in cholesterol; however dietary cholesterol doesn't raise blood cholesterol in most people [157] [158]. This is because the liver produces cholesterol every day and when we eat food containing cholesterol it just produces less [159]. The liver makes cholesterol because it's essential: cholesterol makes many of our hormones, such as testosterone and oestrogen. All our cell membranes use it, and it's necessary for the conversion process to turn sunlight into a usable form of vitamin D that helps to keep our bones strong and our immune systems healthy.

Cholesterol is the name for a family of proteins, including HDL (high-density lipoprotein) and LDL (low-density lipoprotein). HDL is the so-called 'good' cholesterol. It scavenges the bloodstream picking up bits of LDL cholesterol that shouldn't be there.

LDL is the so-called 'bad' cholesterol. Many people don't know that LDL is also an umbrella term for several different-sized particles. Large LDL particles are light and fluffy and don't cause any harm, but low-density particles are very small, dense, and heavy. Scientists believe that these are the particles that contribute to atherosclerosis and heart disease [160]. When people eat eggs, the HDL cholesterol increases [161].

There is now a recognition that eggs should be part of a healthy eating pattern and there is no reason to restrict them in the diet [162] [163].

Replacing the Nutrients in Eggs

If you know you react to eggs and want to exclude them for a while, make sure you aren't missing any nutrients. See the full list of Vitamins, Minerals, and Other Nutrients in Part V: Helpful Resources so that you know what to substitute.

Egg Allergy

Either the proteins in the white of the egg or the yolk can cause an allergy (egg white allergy is more common than yolk allergy). However, there is no safe way to separate the two so if you have an allergy to any part of an egg, you should avoid all of it [164]. It's essential to know which egg proteins cause the allergy as ovalbumin and ovomucin can be broken down by heat so sometimes people can tolerate cooked eggs. Ovomucoid isn't broken down by heat so would still cause an allergic reaction.

Top Tips: if you are sensitive to eggs, look out for these foods:

Albumin, apovitellin, cholesterol free egg substitute (despite the name, this does contain egg white), dried egg solids, dried egg, egg, egg white, egg yolk, egg wash, eggnog. Fat substitutes, globulin, livetin (the protein from egg yolk) and lysozyme (an enzyme found in large quantities in egg white).

Also look out for mayonnaise, meringue, meringue powder, ovalbumin, ovomucin and ovomucoid (the proteins in egg white), ovotransferrin, ovovitellin or vitellin (a protein found in egg yolk), powdered eggs, and silici albuminate, Simplesse (a whey protein concentrate used as a fat replacement in low-calorie foods), Surimi (a paste made from fish or meat and used in Asian cuisines) and whole egg.

Top Tips: these products may contain eggs:

Bakery goods, breaded foods, foam on alcoholic speciality coffees, icings (frostings), marshmallows, mayonnaise, meringue, marzipan, processed meats, meatloaf and meatballs, puddings and custards, salad dressing, many kinds of pasta, and pretzels [165].

Filaggrin Gene Mutation

See earlier for the connection between mutations in the filaggrin gene and allergies to egg, fish, milk and wheat and sensitivity to alcohol.

Anyone with an egg allergy should avoid vaccines for some nasal-spray flu vaccines and yellow fever vaccine as they can contain egg [166].

Fish (This is a Top 14 Allergen)

More than 3.1 billion people in the world depend on fish for at least 20% of their animal protein intake. A further 1.3 billion people rely on fish for 15% of their animal protein intake. Fish consumption has increased from 9 kg per capita in 1961 to approximately 20 kg per capita today and is expected to reach 21.5 kg by 2024 [167].

Health Benefits of Fish

Oily fish are a fantastic source of omega-3 fats. These oils improve mood and cognition, give us cardiovascular benefits, joint protection, support eye health and decrease cancer risk. Oily fish are salmon, mackerel, anchovies, sardines and herring. Other fish have additional benefits in giving us energy and helping us sleep.

The Nutritional Profile of Fish

Fish contain reasonable levels of calcium choline, folate, iodine, selenium, potassium, phosphorous, tryptophan, vitamins B2, B3, B5, B6, B12, D, E and omega-3 fats.

While most people with a fish allergy are allergic to several types of fish, this isn't always the case. Fish is very nutritious, so it's helpful to know which fish is causing a problem so that you don't exclude foods unnecessarily. An allergy test will help identify this (see Part III: Tests). You don't have to eat fish for symptoms to occur. Some people can react to the steam that comes from cooking a fish or from touching it.

Fish Allergy

Usually, this is an allergy to a protein in finned fish called parvalbumin, but it could also be an allergy to the gelatine and bones of the fish [168]. Parvalbumins are found in high quantity in the white muscle tissue of fish, whereas there is much less of the allergen in red muscle tissues. Fish such as tuna have mostly red muscle tissue, and these are often better tolerated by people who are allergic to fish [169]. Cooking doesn't destroy parvalbumins. Both raw and cooked fish can trigger symptoms.

Fish allergy symptoms are:

Anaphylaxis (less common), asthma, diarrhoea, hives or a skin rash, headaches, indigestion, nausea, sneezing, stomach cramps, a stuffy or a runny nose and vomiting.

Top Tips: if you are sensitive to fish, look out for these foods:

Anchovies, bass, cod, flounder, grouper, haddock, hake, halibut, herring, mahi-mahi, perch, pike, pollock, salmon, swordfish, sole, snapper, tilapia, trout and tuna.

Top Tips: these products may contain fish:

Barbecue sauce, bouillabaisse, caponata (a Sicilian aubergine relish), pizzas, relishes, salad dressings, stock cubes, surimi (imitation crab) and Worcestershire sauce. People with a fish allergy may safely consume fish oil supplements as they don't contain fish protein [170].

Fish Allergy and Alcohol

I want to take what might seem a slight diversion to talk about alcohol: during the final stages of brewing wine, beer or even juice beverages the brewer adds something called 'finings' to the liquid. Finings are a fine powder that causes the yeast to sink to the bottom of the barrel, leaving clear alcohol. Isinglass (which comes from the dried swim bladders of fish), egg or casein can all be used to make finings.

For those with a fish allergy, there is a minimal risk of reaction with alcohol that has been fined using isinglass. The alcohol on its own may not cause a response, and a small amount of fish on its own may not produce a reaction, but having the two together may be a different story [171].

Also think carefully about eating in African, Chinese, Indonesian, Thai or Vietnamese restaurants. Even if you don't order fish, there is a high risk of cross-contamination in the kitchen and preparation areas.

Fish Cross-Reactivity

There is usually no cross-reactivity between fish and shellfish (crustaceans and molluscs).

Filaggrin Gene Mutation

See earlier for the connection between mutations in the filaggrin gene and allergies to egg, fish, milk, wheat and sensitivity to alcohol.

FODMAPS Foods

The concept of FODMAPS (Fermentable Oligo-Di-Monosaccharides and Polyols) came about through research work done at Monash University in Melbourne, Australia. The researchers discovered that various short-chain sugars have something in common: they aren't absorbed by humans (or aren't absorbed very well). They ferment and then they produce a lot of gas in the small intestine [172]. When these sugars reach the large intestine, they start to draw in water by a process called osmosis [173].

This watery, gassy mixture causes the walls of the intestine to expand and stimulate nerves in the gut [174]. The stimulation results in the type of pain and discomfort typical of 'IBS-D' (IBS with diarrhoea). This connection to certain foods also explains why people who are sensitive to FODMAPS don't have pain and diarrhoea all the time, only when they eat high-FODMAP foods – foods that are high in these various sugars.

A low FODMAP diet [175] may reduce gluten sensitivity and be even more beneficial than a diet that's solely gluten-free.

The symptoms of FODMAPS intolerance may include:

Abdominal pain, bloating, constipation, diarrhoea [176], gas [177] and nausea. There can also be symptoms of fatigue, lethargy and poor concentration.

FODMAPS include:

- Fructose: fruits and honey are the primary sources [178]

- Fructans: these are high in garlic, inulin, onion and wheat

- Galactans: foods such as legumes, e.g. beans, lentils, and soybeans, are high in these

- Polyols: these are in sweeteners containing mannitol, sorbitol, xylitol and stone fruits such as apricots, avocado, cherries, nectarines, peaches, and plums

- Lactose: dairy is the culprit. Lactose deserves a little more discussion due to the genetic connection – see separate section on Lactose.

The Low FODMAPS

The low FODMAPS foods here are tolerated quite well, because they have a smaller quantity of the indigestible sugars, and there are a lot to choose from:

Eggs, Meat, Poultry, and Fish:

Beef, chicken, cod, eggs, fish, haddock, lamb, lobster, mussels, oysters, plaice, pork, prosciutto, Quorn, salmon, shellfish, shrimp, trout, tuna, turkey and seafood such as crab and prawns (if you don't add anything else to them).

Dairy:

Camembert, cheddar, Feta cheese, Havarti cheese, Lactose-free milk products (milk, yoghurt or ice-cream), Mozzarella, parmesan. These have much lower lactose content than cow's milk.

Fruits:

Bananas, bilberries, blueberries, cantaloupe, Galia and honeydew melon, cranberries, clementine, grapes, guava (ripe), kiwi, all citrus fruits, lemon including lemon juice, lime including lime juice, mandarin, orange, passion fruit, papaya, pineapple, raspberries, rhubarb, strawberries and rhubarb.

Grains:

Most gluten-free grains, oats, rice, tapioca and quinoa.

Non-Dairy Alternatives:

Almond, coconut and rice milks (*not* soya), nut butter and tofu.

Vegetables:

Alfalfa, aubergine (eggplant), bamboo shoots, bean sprouts, beetroot canned and pickled, bell pepper, bok choy, broccoli, brussels sprouts, butternut squash, carrots, cabbage, celeriac, celery (less than 5cm of the stalk).

Also chicory leaves, chives, courgettes (zucchini), corn/sweetcorn (small amounts), cucumbers, fennel, ginger, green beans, kale, lettuce, marrow, nori (the seaweed wraps used to make sushi), okra, olives, parsnips, peppers, potatoes, pumpkin, radishes, seaweed, spinach, squash, swede, swiss chard, sweet potato, tomatoes, turnips, and water chestnuts.

Drinks:

Coffee, tea, herbal tea.

Other:

> Butter, chia seed, clover honey, flaxseed, the green part of chives, olives, pepper, pumpkin seeds, salt, sesame seeds, sunflower seeds and vinegar.

High FODMAPS

High FODMAPS foods aren't tolerated well by individuals who have FODMAPS intolerances. These are:

Dairy:

> Buttermilk, cottage cheese, halloumi, ricotta, cream, cream cheese, custard, ice cream, kefir, Mascarpone, milk (cow's milk, goat's milk, evaporated milk, sheep's milk) sour cream, and yoghurt.

Fruits:

> Apples, apricots, bananas, blackberries, blackcurrants, boysenberry, canned fruit, cherries, currants, dates, dried fruit, goji berries, grapefruit, guava, lychee, mango, nectarine, papaya, peaches, pears, persimmon, pineapple, plums, pomegranate, prunes, raisins, sultanas, tinned fruit and watermelon.

Grains:

> Ground almond, amaranth flour, barley including barley flour, bran cereals, bread such as granary bread, multigrain bread, naan, oatmeal bread, pumpernickel bread, chapati, sourdough, cashews, couscous, einkorn flour, gnocchi, granola bar, muesli, pistachios, rye, semolina, spelt flour and wheat.

Non-Dairy Alternatives:

> Beans, bulgur wheat, baked beans, black-eyed beans, butter beans, cashews, haricot beans, kidney beans, lentils, mung beans, miso, pistachios, red kidney beans, soybeans and soy milk and split peas.

Vegetables:

> Artichoke, asparagus, beetroot, broad beans, cassava, cauliflower, celery (greater than 5cm of stalk), garlic, leek, mange

tout, mushrooms, onions, sauerkraut, savoy cabbage, the bulb of spring onions (scallions), shallots, and sugar snap peas.

Drinks:

Beer (if drinking more than one bottle), coconut water, cordial, fruit and herbal teas with apple added, fruit juices made of apple, pear, mango, kombucha, or orange juice in quantities over 100ml. Rum, sodas containing high fructose corn syrup (HFCS). Sports drinks, black tea with added soy milk, chai tea (strong), dandelion tea (strong), fennel tea, chamomile tea, herbal tea (strong), oolong tea, wine (if drinking more than one glass). Soy milk, whey protein, whey concentrate unless lactose-free, whey protein and hydrolysed whey unless lactose-free.

Other:

Agave syrup, caviar dip, fructose, gravy if it contains onion, honey of any kind except clover honey, high fructose corn syrup (HFCS). Jam, pesto sauce, relish or vegetable pickle, sugar-free sweets containing polyols – usually ending in -ol or isomalt, inulin, maltitol, mannitol, sorbitol, stock cubes, xylitol, tahini paste or tzatziki dip.

The Low FODMAP Diet

For those people who are sensitive to FODMAPS, try the low FODMAP diet for six to eight weeks (this means avoiding all the foods that are on the high FODMAPS list just for that period). During this time, the body can heal. Then introduce specific items from the high FODMAP list, one at a time. Allow four days between each introduction to see if the new food causes any symptoms. If a high FODMAP food causes no symptoms, include it in your diet and introduce the next food. Avoid it if it still causes problems.

The diet will be a unique combination of foods for everyone, as some foods will be acceptable and some won't. Sometimes food can be included if it's a low quantity. It isn't necessarily a question of all or nothing but of knowing which foods are high in FODMAPs, which gives you a more sensitive search tool with which to work out what is causing your symptoms [179] [180] [181].

The FODMAPS diet seems to be very useful in dealing with symptoms of IBS [174] and deals with several other conditions such as amines (see below), gluten and salicylates sensitivities [175].

High Histamine Foods

Histamine occurs naturally in foods and is also produced by the body when under stress. It plays a prominent role in the allergy response by sending messages from your body to your brain (already covered in the earlier discussion on allergies).

Histamine is a major cause of inflammation. High-histamine foods can cause inflammation in some people. Storage or maturation conditions play a part in increasing the natural histamine to a level that will prompt a more significant reaction. Foods that are naturally low in histamine will have an increasing level of histamine as the foods age or ripen (for example, leftover beef, or a ripe tomato as opposed to a green one).

Symptoms of Histamine Intolerance

You may notice any of the following:

> Abdominal cramps, arrhythmia or accelerated heart rate, difficulty breathing, difficulty falling asleep or waking up easily, dizziness, difficulty regulating body temperature, fatigue, flushing, headaches or migraines, hives, hypertension, nasal congestion, nausea, sneezing, tissue swelling, vertigo or vomiting.

Foods High in Histamine

Foods high in histamine are:

> Alcohol (acetaldehyde), aubergine (eggplant), bananas, canned fish, cheeses, chocolate, citrus fruits, egg whites, fermented soy, food additives, ketchup, mackerel, nuts, pork, preservatives such as benzoates (BHA and BHT), tartrazine, food colours, sauerkraut, sausage, smoked meats, spinach, strawberries, tomatoes, tuna, vinegar and wheat germ.

Look out for foods that intentionally contain high levels of microbes or introduce microbes as part of the maturation process, such as long-ripened cheese, pickled cabbage and red wine. These will be high in histamine.

Scombroid Poisoning

A further risk area for high histamine is high-protein fish that have been accidentally contaminated with microbes through poor storage or cooking procedures. Saltwater environments readily contain the kinds of bacteria that result in histamine development. The bacteria can be found on the gills, on the external surfaces and in the gut of the fish without causing any ill effects to the creature. The fish has its defence mechanisms to stop the growth of histamine; however, when the fish dies, these defences also die.

Incorrect handling procedures may spread the bacteria from the inside of the fish to the flesh. Processing the fish (butchering or filleting) may also spread the bacteria. It can be particularly problematic for fish with a large volume of muscle tissue, such as tuna. The harvested fish need to be kept at a temperature of 4.4° centigrade (39.92° fahrenheit) or less, as the bacteria is active at just above that figure. It should remain at this temperature until consumption.

Extended frozen storage (up to twenty-four weeks) or cooking disables the bacteria. Canning, salting or vacuum packaging doesn't necessarily inhibit the bacteria [182]. Cooking or a sterilisation process will remove the bacteria but won't remove any existing scombrotoxin (the name for the histamine-releasing toxin). Once a fish is contaminated, the contamination can't be removed. The development of scombrotoxin also involves biogenic amines (mentioned below).

Histamine levels in canned tuna are typically in the range of 1 ppm (part per million) to 30 ppm. It's perfectly safe to consume. Food regulations in most countries allow a histamine range of up to 100 ppm. In some cases where there is a flawed supply chain, the fish isn't chilled correctly, or there is inadequate hygiene with fish kept in the open air in tropical temperatures, high histamine levels of 200 ppm to 500 ppm can develop [183].

73

Increased Likelihood of Reactions to Histamine

Chronic diseases such as kidney disease (renal insufficiency), various medications (aspirin, non-steroidal anti-inflammatory drugs - NSAIDs, medicines used during x-rays, and opiates such as codeine or morphine) increase the likelihood of reactions to high levels of histamine.

Top Tip:
> If you are sensitive to histamine, eat food that's freshly prepared and freeze any leftover foods (particularly those containing protein) as soon as possible.

Biogenic Amines

The enzymes that break down histamine also break down chemicals called biogenic amines very quickly. Usually, people can tolerate small quantities of amines. Some drugs inhibit this breakdown:
> Antibiotics (amoxicillin/clavulanic acid, doxycycline, isoniazid), metoclopramide, verapamil, promethazine and older antidepressants (monoamine oxidase inhibitors)

The most common symptoms experienced are eczema, fatigue (feeling very tired for no reason), diarrhoea or constipation, hives, headaches, joint pain, migraines, mouth ulcers, nausea, or sinus problems. Children can become irritable, restless, or show symptoms related to ADHD. If the mother has many amines in her diet, breastfed babies may experience colic, eczema, loose stools, and nappy (diaper) rash.

Lectins

Lectins are a family of carbohydrate-binding proteins found everywhere in nature. Legumes, grains, dairy, seafood, and nightshades (see Nightshades section) contain the most lectins. Nightshade plants are potatoes, aubergine (eggplant), tomatoes and peppers. Several nightshade spices also contain lectins: cayenne, chilli, and paprika.
Plants produce lectins to protect themselves from being eaten. The lectins make molecules stick together. In your own body, lectins are involved in the immune system by recognising carbohydrates that don't belong, but they can wreak havoc if you don't have the enzymes to digest

them [184]. Then they can set off allergic reactions that weaken the gut lining and allow it to become leaky.

Lectins are highly resistant to being broken down in the stomach and can pass through it unchanged. The digestive and nervous systems are particularly sensitive to lectin reactions. Lectin symptoms can appear as IBS, arthritis or nearly any inflammatory condition [185].

The Science Behind Lectins

When food travels through your gut, it causes minor damage to the gut wall. Your body repairs this quite easily and quickly, but lectins slow down this repair, and this can result in intestinal permeability. Lectins interfere with the enterocytes (cells on top of the intestinal 'carpet') and lymphocytes (a type of cell in the immune system).

The gut isn't the only place for immune system activation. It occurs throughout the body and can result in the immune system attacking peripheral tissues through a process called 'molecular mimicry'. As lectins are sticky, they bind to cell surfaces in the body and become a new biochemical compound including the cell they attach to.

Antibodies are initially created as 'blanks'. They're subsequently trained to recognise just one foreign substance. Antibodies that learn lectins as a foreign substance can be confused by the new biochemical compound. It contains the lectin and so must be treated as 'foreign', even though a part of it is your own body. The immune system then attacks 'self' (a term which means your own body). This antibody response can lead to autoimmune and inflammatory conditions such as rheumatoid arthritis [186] [187]. Autoimmunity can have a range of causes, certainly not just lectins.

People with Crohn's disease or IBS seem to have a more sensitive gut lining that can react to lectins.

Should You Avoid Lectins?

Almost all foods contain lectins to some degree. Never eat raw legumes and lectins as they're poisonous in this state. When eaten raw, the lectins can result in nausea, diarrhoea, and vomiting. However, you can neutralise lectins contained in food with the correct preparation – this means soaking and boiling the beans before eating them [188]. See Part IV: Solutions - Increasing Nutrient Power and Reducing Lectins.

How Long Do Lectin Problems Last?

The effects of lectins only last for the time that they're in the body, which is thought to be around twenty-four hours. Any symptoms can be reduced by eating a varied diet with plenty of fruit and vegetables, as these foods will nourish your 'friendly' gut bacteria and these, in turn, will look after your gut.

Don't use raw legume flours in baked goods as lectins are resistant to dry heat.

There is another downside to lectins – they do cause flatulence! This can be reduced by cooking them with a pinch of a spice called asafoetida which is available online.

Ricin

To illustrate how strong lectins *can* be: you may have heard of the poison, 'Ricin'. It has nothing to do with rice. It's a highly toxic lectin found in the seeds of the castor oil plant, Ricinus communis. A lethal dose of purified ricin powder is only the size of a few grains of table salt. If you are searching your memory for the reason why you remember this lectin, you may remember the murder of Georgi Markov. He was a Bulgarian dissident living in London in 1978. Someone murdered him with a pellet of ricin fired into his leg from a specially-adapted umbrella.

Legumes

Legumes are a class of vegetables that include lentils, beans and peas. Although peanuts and soy are part of the same family, they have separate sections in this book because individually they're in the Top 14 Allergens list.

Legumes are among the most nutritious foods available. They were first cultivated in the bronze age (from about 2500 B.C. to 800 B.C.). Ancient Egyptians considered beans to be an emblem of life and had temples dedicated to them. The Romans' four most distinguished families were named after beans - Fabius (fava bean), Lentulus (lentil), Piso (pea), and Cicero (chickpea).

Health Benefits of Legumes

Legumes are typically low in fat and are high in folate, calcium, phosphorous, potassium, iron, zinc and magnesium [189]. They're high in soluble and insoluble fibre and also contain beneficial fats [190]. At a small fraction of the cost of meat protein, one cup of cooked beans provides 25% of the daily requirement for the amino acids [191]. The legume family consists of many different types of bean, all with slightly different nutritional profiles. It's good to include a selection of them in your diet.

Legumes Intolerances and Allergies

Legumes can trigger significant allergic reactions. Symptoms can include eczema and hives, nasal congestion and asthma, difficulty breathing and a feeling of tightness in the chest and anaphylaxis. There is a high degree of allergenic cross-reactivity among different members of the legume family [192].

Any of these could be intolerance symptoms:

Acne, bloating, eczema, headaches and migraines, IBS, itchy skin, respiratory problems such as a runny nose, tiredness and fatigue.

Chickpeas (garbanzo beans) are high FODMAP foods – see section on FODMAPS.

Lupin (This is a Top 14 Allergen)

The lupin family contains over 200 different species. In Europe, white lupin beans from the species L.Albus are eaten whole as a pickled snack food. L. Angustifolius (narrow-leafed lupin) and L. Hirsutus (blue lupin) are also edible. Lupin seeds are ground into flour for gluten-free goods.

Lupini dishes are found mostly in Europe: in Greece, Portugal, Spain and Italy. In Israel, Jordan, Lebanon and Syria they're served as an appetiser.

They're also eaten in Brazil and Egypt. Most lupin seeds go to make animal feed, but there is a growing recognition that they can also be used for human food as an alternative to soya. About 85% of the world's lupin seeds are grown in Western Australia [193].

Manufacturers introduced lupin flour to the UK as a food ingredient in 1996 and France in 1997. It's very high in protein (30%-40%) and dietary fibre (40%), and it comes from the same botanical group as peanuts (i.e. the legumes family). People who have an allergy to peanuts can have an allergy to lupin as well [194]. Eating or inhaling lupin can trigger the allergy.

Lupin flour can make up 20% of the volume of wheat-based products [195] and up to 50% of the volume of biscuits. Pasta, sauces, and beverages also use lupin, and the proteins aren't broken down by heating.

Lupin Symptoms

The symptoms of a mild lupin allergy are a tingling or itchy feeling in the mouth, or hives, which can be anywhere on the body. More severe symptoms are uncommon in the UK because lupin is only used in small quantities, but may extend to anaphylactic shock.

Top Tips: if you are sensitive to lupin, look out for these foods -
Lupin or lupine, lupin flour, lupin seed, and lupin bean.

Top Tips: these products may contain lupin -
Crepes, deep-coated vegetables such as onion rings, pancakes, pastry cases, pies, pizzas, products containing crumb, vegetarian meat substitute and waffles.

Milk (This is a Top 14 Allergen)

All types of dairy milk fall into this classification of a Top 14 allergen, whether they're from cows, goats or sheep, and whether they're full-fat, semi-skimmed, skimmed, low-fat, UHT or any other variation.

Does everyone in the world drink milk? There are distinct regions of milk drinkers. The populations of northern and central European descent love milk (this extends to all the places that Europeans colonised historically). In southern and eastern Europe, there are some milk drinkers and some non-milk drinkers. Africa and the Middle East show a more complex pattern with people who herd cattle often drinking milk but with it being much less commonplace in their non-herding neighbours. People of Asian descent don't generally drink milk [196].

Germany and France are the top two milk producers in Europe. The UK is the tenth-largest producer in the world. Milk accounted for 17.8% of total agricultural output in the UK in 2014 and was worth £4.6bn in market prices.

The total number of UK dairy cows has fallen from 2.6 million in 1996 to 1.9 million in 2015, a 27% reduction, and yet, despite this, the UK produced 14.6 billion litres of milk in 2014, the highest annual figure since 1990 [197].

Dairy farming has become much more intensive with breeds such as the Holstein-Friesian producing up to 60 litres of milk per day [198]. The European Union banned the use of artificial growth hormone (bovine somatotropin) in 2000 although this is still legal in the US [199]. At the same time, the European Union also banned imports of milk from cows treated with bovine somatotropin [200], which means European countries can't import any milk from the US.

Issues with milk can be caused by two factors [201]:

- Lactose (the sugar in milk – see the science of lactose, below), which needs the enzyme lactase to break it down (this is an *intolerance*);

- Milk protein, usually casein (this is a *sensitivity*).

Do We Need Milk?

I'm going to be controversial here and say that there is no need for humans to drink milk past weaning. We are the only animal that ingests the milk of another animal. When children drink milk, it makes them

79

grow because it's a perfect growth food – but it's a perfect food for calves, not children.

The perfect food for babies is human breast milk. When we are no longer babies, we don't need it, and we have a choice whether we consume it or not. There are several reasons why it may be better not to have too much cow's milk:

- The nutrients are present in different proportions from human milk;

- The nutrients in cow's milk are specifically designed to enable a calf to grow into a large cow in just two years. Part of the reason for this is the higher proportion of fat in cow's milk. Humans generally don't stop developing until they're between fifteen and seventeen years old. Our human growth rate is much slower. We don't need to drink something that attempts to accelerate that growth rate;

- Cow's milk is an easy source of many good nutrients. This is often one of the arguments in its favour. However, we shouldn't drink milk in preference to eating a balanced diet containing a good range of nutrients, as we miss out on all the other food benefits that are available to us (other nutrients, fibre and more);

- The size of the protein molecules in milk is different; cows are very large animals and produce large proteins. Our bodies regard these as foreign, as indeed they are. Humans, in comparison, produce smaller proteins in their milk. The large proteins can contribute to sensitivity to the casein (the major protein in milk) – see later;

- Cow's milk is higher in calcium than human milk. Yes, as adults, we still need sufficient calcium, but we can get plenty of calcium in other foods such as sardines, spinach, kale, shellfish, and tofu [202]. Surely, it's an advantage to have more calcium? Not necessarily. Too much of something isn't necessarily a good thing, as the following study shows:

80

- A 2005 study investigating the rate of osteoporosis in the elderly after consuming a high-calcium diet for most of their lives found that increased calcium intake 'wore out' the cells responsible for renewing bone (called osteoblasts). Instead of being *protective* against osteoporosis, the calcium was *contributing* to it, as old bone was broken down more than new bone was built to replace it [203];

- Regularly drinking cow's milk has been associated with many health risks, including prostate and ovarian cancers, autoimmune diseases, and some childhood illnesses [204] [205] [206];

- Cow's milk naturally contains an opioid chemical that affects our brain chemistry, making us want to drink more (more on this later).

If you really want cow's milk in your morning tea or coffee, and nothing else will do, then enjoy it, but be mindful that a lot of health conditions are associated with dairy, and for some people, the tolerance or sensitivity threshold is incredibly low. It isn't food that you *must* consume.

While cow's milk has a lot of potential issues for all ages, cheese and yoghurt can be better choices. At least these are fermented (more on this later) so that they reduce food intolerance problems and retain nutrients.

Cheese and yoghurt are also practical and cost-effective solutions for children whose tastebuds aren't too receptive to the bitter flavours of kale and spinach or other calcium-rich alternatives.

Milk and Bones

The most significant indicator of the health and strength of our bones in later life isn't how much milk we drank, but our peak bone mass density at around the age of 30. After this, bone density naturally starts to decline. All through our lives we are making new bone and breaking down old bone. When these two processes are in balance, we have healthy bones.

81

One of the critical factors in achieving good bone mass density is weight-bearing exercise. However, we need more than this. We also need proper protein intake and adequate vitamin D, as well as calcium. Calcium metabolism also has a counter-intuitive feature – the more we take in, the less we absorb [207] [208] [209].

Falls and bone fracture rates in the elderly are related to low vitamin D levels, as vitamin D controls whether calcium is deposited in bones and in what quantity [210]. We also need something called parathyroid hormone to be doing its job correctly (it regulates calcium levels in the blood). As you can see, the situation isn't as simple as: "drink milk and all will be well."

Nutritional Profile of Milk

Milk contains the following nutrients at high levels:

> Calcium, phosphorous, iodine, magnesium, vitamins A, B1, B2, B12, and zinc. The US fortifies milk with vitamin D, but it isn't enriched in the UK.

The Science of Lactose

Lactose is a sugar found in milk. It's called a disaccharide because it's a compound made up of one part of galactose and one part of glucose. It's digested (broken down) by an enzyme called lactase in the small intestine. Once broken down, its two constituent parts are known as monosaccharides. They can be absorbed through the gut into our bloodstream and then transported around the body so that our cells can use them for fuel. If we don't need more energy at the time they're absorbed, sugars transform into fats for storage.

Our bodies are incredibly efficient; they only produce whatever materials are deemed necessary. The instructions to do this come from our genes; our DNA. The usual state for all mammals is that milk is food for the newborn only for the first few months of life. As far as Mother Nature is concerned when we start to eat solid foods we no longer need milk. At this time, our bodies reduce the production of the enzyme to break down lactose (you may remember, the enzyme is called lactase).

Production of lactase starts to diminish at around the age of two or three and stops almost entirely between the age of five to ten. When we don't produce the lactase enzyme, we can't break down lactose. We may be able to tolerate a tiny amount of it [211], but any more gives us a problem.

A 2016 study published in the journal Nutrients showed that lactose-intolerant people could consume up to twelve grams of lactose at a time without symptoms – this is the amount of lactose in a whole cup of milk (8 fl. oz or 250 ml) [212]. I find this very surprising as the experience of my clients suggests that they couldn't tolerate anything like this amount. However, this does raise a question for all those who suffer from vague digestive discomfort and loose bowels sometimes and can't isolate the cause. Everyone's tolerance level is different. People can still be lactose-intolerant while being able to drink a small amount of milk, apparently without symptoms.

These issues are called 'lactase non-persistence.' This genetic trait is common around the world, but particularly in people with African and Asian ancestry.

Lactose and DNA

When domestication of dairy animals began, humans realised that drinking their milk could be a source of nutrition. Over time, for those populations herding animals, DNA mutated to allow them to continue producing lactase and therefore able to digest the milk of another mammal. The same gene mutation happened in many different places around the world simultaneously [213].

Can we work out exactly when this happened? Some scientists have tried. They took DNA from ten skeletons: One was around 2,300 years old. Eight were between 5,000-6,000 years old, and one was 500 years old. Of these, only the 500-year-old skeleton showed lactose tolerance. All the others showed lactose intolerance in their DNA.

Although this was just a small sample, it gives us an idea of how lactose tolerance might have developed. It wasn't common 5,000 years ago, but there are indications that people were drinking milk 500 years ago[214] [215].

Types of Lactose Intolerance

There are three types of lactose intolerance:

- Primary lactose intolerance: the gene switches off during childhood, and this condition is lifelong;

- Secondary lactose intolerance: conditions affecting the small intestine (such as inflammation or infection) affect the production of the lactase enzyme temporarily, and this can be resolved;

- Congenital lactose intolerance: (very rare) the person has never been able to produce lactase.

A few thousand years ago a genetic mutation appeared in the lactase gene in central Europe, which meant that the gene stayed active all through life – creating lactose persistence. After a few generations it became common as dairy became an increasingly important part of the central European diet, so now some people *are* tolerant to lactose [216].

The Proteins in Cow's Milk

Roughly 80% of cow's milk proteins are casein with 20% being whey. Casein itself is made up of 13 different proteins; the most common are A1 beta-casein and A2 beta-casein:

- A1 milk contains both A1 beta-casein and A2 beta-casein and comes from Holstein, Friesian, Ayrshire and British Shorthorn cows. Almost all the supermarket milk that we buy is A1 milk. It doesn't have a label of A1 milk, but we know it as whole milk (or full-fat milk), semi-skimmed milk or skimmed milk;

- A2 milk contains just A2 beta-casein and comes from older breeds that originated in the Channel Islands and Southern France. These breeds include the Guernsey, Jersey, Charolais and Limousin. In some larger shops, you may see a type of milk called 'A2 Milk,' although it isn't very commonly available. It comes from the older breeds mentioned above.

The Science Behind the Breakdown of Beta-Caseins

The A2 breeds produce a chemical called proline alongside the casein in their milk. Proline binds strongly to another chemical called BCM-7 (beta-casomorphin 7). This bond stops the BCM-7 getting into the guts of the cows and from there getting into the A2 milk. A2 milk is virtually BCM-7-free.

The newer breeds of cows (such as Friesian) make a different bond with BCM-7 using a chemical called histidine. Histidine forms a weak bond with BCM-7, which breaks easily. BCM-7 is released in the guts of cows and finds its way into their milk. Why am I making a fuss about BCM-7? It's an opioid. Opioids bind to specific receptors in the brain and in the rest of the body which control pain, digestion and affect the brain's pleasure (reward) centre.

Some people can break down BCM-7 rapidly, in which case it doesn't cause problems, but those who can't break it down may experience inflammatory reactions anywhere in the body. There is also a human form of BCM-7 in breast milk, but its chemical structure is entirely different, and it works in our bodies differently.

BCM-7 in the gut can produce both IgE and IgG antibody responses. BCM-7 increases mucus production in the gut, and this can interfere with our 'friendly' bacteria [217] [218] [219] [220], and consequently interfere with the nourishment our body receives.

Issues Associated with Cow's Milk

A1 casein can create a wide range of problems in addition to digestive problems: everything from heart disease to Type 1 diabetes, autism to schizophrenia and neurodevelopmental delay in children [221] [222] [223] [224] [225].

If you have issues due to A1 casein, you may experience symptoms such as brain fog and lethargy, digestive symptoms of bloating and diarrhoea, or excess mucus production, which can affect the sinuses, ears, throat or bowels [226] [227].

While A1 beta-casein seems a common culprit, there have been immune reactions to other proteins [228].

Top Tips: if you are sensitive to milk, look out for these foods -
Cheese, cream, chocolate, custard, instant mash, milk, margarine, milk powder, butter, buttermilk, caramel flavouring, flavouring, ghee, high protein flour, ice cream, lactic acid starter culture, natural flavouring, rice cheese, soy cheese and yoghurt.

Top Tips: any of these products could contain milk -
Dairy products such as butter, cheese, cream, milk powders and yoghurt. Milk is a favourite glaze to put on foods. It's also commonly found in powdered soups and sauces.

The Size of the Problem: Working Through the Dairy Families

When I carry out a food intolerance test, I'm often asked why there can be a difference in response to cow's milk and goat's milk, or why cheese or yoghurt may not provoke a reaction when milk does. The best way to explain this is, firstly, to think of the size of the animal. The smaller the animal, the smaller the protein. Goats are smaller than cows, so their proteins are smaller. Sheep are smaller than goats, so their proteins are the smallest. We break down smaller proteins more easily.

The second factor is the level of fermentation. Fermentation is a process that breaks down proteins and sugars. Milk contains proteins (caseins), and the sugar is lactose. Cheese is more fermented than milk and is easier to digest [229] [230]. Yoghurt is more fermented than cheese. Yoghurt causes the least reaction.

Most lactose-intolerant people can tolerate butter as it contains only trace amounts of lactose. Butter contains 1% protein (the casein) [231], and most people who are sensitive to casein can tolerate this too. If you have a strong allergy to milk protein then you should still avoid butter as the tiniest amount of the protein could result in a strong allergic reaction.

Ghee is purely fat and all people should be able to tolerate it.

The following table explains it:

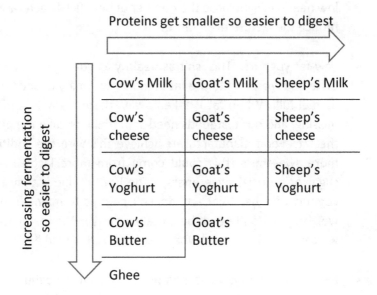

Proteins get smaller so easier to digest →		
Cow's Milk	Goat's Milk	Sheep's Milk
Cow's cheese	Goat's cheese	Sheep's cheese
Cow's Yoghurt	Goat's Yoghurt	Sheep's Yoghurt
Cow's Butter	Goat's Butter	
Ghee		

Increasing fermentation so easier to digest ↓

Yoghurt and Lactose

According to the Dairy Council, a staggering 91.6% of UK households bought yoghurt in 2015, and since the 1970s yoghurt consumption in the UK has increased by a massive 340% [232]. Yoghurt is naturally low in lactose and may be beneficial for those who are lactose intolerant [233]. Yoghurt is even more fermented than cheese, and so the sugars are further broken down. All yoghurt contains some level of bacteria. There are four varieties:

- Greek yoghurt. This is very thick and creamy, but it tastes tart because it's low in lactose. (As a sugar, lactose tastes sweet);

- Live or Active yoghurt. The active part is bacteria called Lactobacillus bulgaricus and Streptococcus thermophilus. They feed on the lactose to break it down, doing the work for you. This is easier to digest;

- Full-fat yoghurt, which is lower in lactose than low-fat yoghurts. You can also make home-made full-fat yoghurt very easily. If you heat it for longer than the usual manufacturer's eight hours on low heat you'll increase the number of beneficial bacteria and so reduce the lactose even more;

- Low-fat yoghurt. This isn't as healthy as you might think. Our taste buds respond to the fat in food – we enjoy it, and it makes us feel full. When fat is taken away, there really is something missing, and our tastebuds need something to take the place of the fat. Food manufacturers achieve this with the addition of more sweetness (this could come from more lactose, added sugar or artificial sweeteners). The bottom line is that low-fat yoghurt isn't healthier and doesn't help us to maintain or lose weight. We don't need the fat taken away in the first place, and we certainly don't need what is substituted. Avoid it;

- Fermented and unsweetened products such as yoghurt contain natural bacteria that make it easier to digest. We don't know whether yoghurt contains BCM-7 [230].

Butter

Butter contains very little lactose (even less than yoghurt). Also, it has very little protein - that results in very little whey or casein and less likelihood of an intolerance reaction. Ghee is butter that has been 'clarified', which means it has been heated to separate the proteins from the fat. The proteins float on the surface of the hot fat and can be removed. The remaining soft fat is ghee, with no protein and no sugar (lactose). Intolerance reactions are caused by proteins. Ghee is 100% fat with no protein so doesn't cause intolerance reactions.

What to look for on the label

If it were just the word 'milk' on the label, it would be so easy to avoid it! Unfortunately, this is one product where there are many variations:

Any term including the words milk or buttermilk (acidophilus, blend, condensed, cow's, cultured, dry milk solids DMS. Solids, evaporated, fat, fat-free, full cream, goat's, lactose-free, low fat, malted, non-fat. Powder milk derivative, powder, protein, solids, solid pastes, non-fat milk solids, pasteurised, powdered. Sheep's, skimmed, sour, sweet cream, and buttermilk powder, whole, 1%, 2%).

Butter — artificial butter, artificial butter flavour, butter extract, butter fat, butter flavoured oil, butter solids, dairy butter, natural butter, natural butter flavour and whipped butter.

Casein & caseinates — ammonium caseinate, calcium caseinate, hydrolysed casein, iron caseinate, magnesium caseinate, potassium caseinate, sodium caseinate, and zinc caseinate.

Cheese — cheese (all types dairy), cheese flavour (artificial and natural), cheese food, cottage cheese, cream cheese, imitation cheese, vegetarian cheeses with casein.

Cream, whipped cream, curds, custard, dairy product solids, galactose, half & half, sour.

Hydrolysates — casein hydrolysate, milk protein hydrolysate, protein hydrolysate, whey hydrolysate, whey protein hydrolysate, ice cream and ice milk.

Sherbet, casein, whey, lactulose, lactoferrin, lactoglobulin, lactalbumin, lactalbumin phosphate, lactate solids, lactyc yeast, lactitol monohydrate and lactoglobulin.

Lactose, nisin preparation (food preservative), nougat, pudding, quark, recaldent (used in dentistry), rennet, rennet casein and simplesse® (fat replacer).

Any term including the word whey — acid, cured, de-lactosed, demineralised, hydrolysed, powdered, reduced mineral, sweet dairy, protein, powder, and solids.

Yoghurt, and yoghurt powder.

Goat's Milk

Although it isn't as popular in the west, the rest of the world loves goat's milk. Goat's milk is easier to digest for several reasons:

- Goat's milk is lower in lactose (approximately 3.9% in goat's milk compared to 33.7% in cow's milk);

- Although the fat content of cow's and goat's milk is similar, the fat molecules in goat's milk are smaller, with a softer curd that's easier for digestive enzymes to break down. Cow's milk contains agglutinin, which is what makes the fat rise to the top of the liquid. The fat sticks together, making the milk harder to digest. Goat's milk doesn't contain agglutinin and has an even distribution of the fat molecules throughout the milk which makes it easier to digest;

- In the world of biochemistry, size matters for all sorts of reasons. Goat's milk has higher levels of short- and medium-chain fatty acids, making it easier to break down as there are only a few links in the chain of molecules. (Cow's milk contains long chains of molecules, which take more work for your body to break down);

- Goat's milk contains only trace amounts of the allergenic casein protein, A1 beta-casein, found in cow's milk [234] [201] [235].

The Nutritional Profile of Goat's Milk

Goat's milk contains:

Calcium, copper, magnesium, phosphorous, potassium, zinc, vitamins, A, B2, C and D.

Sheep's Milk Cheese

Sheep's cheese is an excellent alternative to cow's cheese and more tolerable for many. The proteins in the cheese are easier to digest in a similar way to goat's cheese.

Top Tips: if you are sensitive to cow's cheese, any of these goat's and sheep's cheeses may be more tolerable -

Feta, Manchego, Pecorino, Ricotta, and Roquefort, but always check the label as sometimes these cheeses include cow's milk to make them cheaper to produce.

Filaggrin Gene Mutation

See earlier for the connection between mutations in the filaggrin gene and allergies to egg, fish, milk, wheat, and sensitivity to alcohol.

Molluscs (These are Top 14 Allergens)

Molluscs are foods such as mussels and snails. They have a hard shell with a soft body and no spine. They have very elaborate nervous systems, which are very different from vertebrate animals such as humans. Some molluscs have clusters of brain cells (called ganglions) rather than actual brains, and some molluscs have brains around their oesphagi. An octopus has its brain cells in its arms, which can function independently even when separated from its body!

The Benefits of Molluscs

Molluscs provide healthy vitamins and minerals, particularly vitamin B12. They're low in fat and high in omega-3 fats. Molluscs have many health benefits, including keeping the heart healthy and fighting arthritis and joint pain (glucosamine comes from molluscs). They help the circulatory system, the immune system and improve fertility. They're a good source of iron and so can assist in preventing anaemia. Skin care, healthy ageing and healthy cellular functions all benefit from the health qualities of molluscs [236].

The Nutritional Profile of Molluscs

Molluscs contain calcium, copper, iron, magnesium, manganese, phosphorous, potassium, selenium, sodium, zinc, vitamins A, B6, B12 and E.

Mollusc Cross-Reactivity

People who have allergic responses to one type of mollusc will very often be allergic to others. They can also react to crustaceans (such as crabs, prawns, and shrimp) and have related allergies to house-dust mite and cockroaches. Shellfish retain their allergic potential even after cooking [237]. Allergic reactions to snails frequently involve asthma [238].

Top Tips: if you are sensitive to molluscs, look out for these foods -
Abalone, clams, cockles, mussels, scallops, snails, octopus, oysters, squid and whelks.

Top Tips: any of these products may contain molluscs -
Calamari, Chinese dim sum, soup and rice porridge, mussel dishes, oyster sauce, sauces, scallops and soups which may contain molluscs.

Mustard (This is a Top 14 Allergen)

Sanskrit writings mentioned mustard about five thousand years ago. The first medicinal reference comes from Hippocrates, who wrote about it being used for general muscular relief. The Romans used it as a condiment and pickling spice, and King Louis XI of France (1423-1483) would travel with his royal mustard pot, in case his hosts didn't serve it [239].

The Health Benefits of Mustard

Mustard has laxative, antibacterial, antifungal, antiseptic and anti-inflammatory properties. It's also a topical treatment for rheumatism and arthritis and can be used to bathe aching feet. It has been used in the form of plasters over the back and chest to treat bronchitis and pneumonia. Internally, mustard seeds can be appetite stimulants, emetics (medicine which induces vomiting) and diuretics (drugs designed to increase urination).

The Nutritional Profile of Mustard

Mustard seeds contain good levels of copper, magnesium, manganese, omega-3 fats, phosphorous, selenium and vitamin B1.

All parts of the mustard plant are likely to cause an allergic reaction in people with a mustard allergy. People who have asthma – especially if poorly controlled – are more likely to have an allergy to mustard.

Top Tips: if you are sensitive to mustard, look out for these foods - Mustard powder, mustard seeds, mustard flour, mustard leaves, mustard oil, sprouted mustard seeds.

Top Tips: look out for these products which may contain mustard - Béarnaise Sauce, BBQ sauce, curry sauce, chutneys, Cumberland sauce, dehydrated soups, fish paste, flavouring or seasoning, gravies, Indian foods (mustard seed or mustard oil). Ketchup, marinades, mayonnaise, pesto, pizza, piccalilli, pickles and pickled products, salad dressing (vinaigrettes and crudités), sausages and processed meat products, Russian foods, sauces, spices, tomato sauce, vegetables with vinegar. In Italy mustard is used to make a sweet mustard syrup with fruits to eat as a relish with meats (look out for the word mostarda).

Mustard Cross-Reactivity

Mustard shows cross-reactivity with mugwort pollen [241] (see later section on Oral Allergy Syndrome).

Medications and Supplements

It may seem odd to include medicine and nutritional supplements in a list of foods, but we do swallow them and digest them. I'm not going to go into whether you should take medication or not – that's a conversation for you to have with your doctor. If you've been prescribed a medicine for a long time, it's always worth checking that you understand why you are taking it and that it's still necessary - you can make an appointment with your doctor for a medication review.

The thing that *does* interest me is investigating the other ingredients contained in the medication or supplement alongside the active ingredients. Manufacturers identify components in the patient information leaflets included with all medication. While patients sometimes read dosage and side-effects (women more than men), few people read the contraindications section that contains this information as they think their doctor told them all they need to know.

However, the same information is often not repeated in the doctor's reference material [242]. Supplements include this information on the side of the container. It usually doesn't get a second glance. I always check medications and supplements for my clients – both the ones that they're already taking and ones that I may recommend. I check that they'll work together, but I also check the excipients for magnesium stearate.

Magnesium Stearate

There are a few things to note concerning excipients. These are substances that are included alongside the active ingredients to bulk-up and stabilise the formulations and, in some cases, make them flow more easily through the factory machinery. They don't do anything for you. The argument goes that because they're present in such small quantities, they don't cause any problems.

The one that gets the most attention is called magnesium stearate (sometimes also called vegetable stearate or stearic acid). This substance - present in minute quantities – really polarises opinion. There are those who say it's entirely safe and there are those who say it's an altogether unnecessary additive with no benefits and lots of drawbacks.

I started to test magnesium stearate when clients came to me with a bag full of supplements that they were taking, either recommended by someone else or bought based on their research. Fiona was such a case. She wanted to know whether her supplements were helping her. In some ways, this seems a strange question to ask – why would you keep taking a supplement if it didn't help?

When people are very ill with several food intolerances on top of other long-standing medical conditions, the body can take its time to respond to anything, and the immediate cause and effect relationship that you might expect to see is just not there. Some days you might feel a bit better, some days you might feel worse, without being able to pinpoint why. Several of Fiona's supplements were helpful to her, but quite a few weren't.

Sometimes supplements don't help because they're just the wrong supplements for the intended purpose. A client may have seen some

94

advertising that a particular supplement was good for energy support, for example, but their energy problem needs a different kind of support, and so the supplement doesn't help them. In this case, Fiona had the right ideas about what might need support. I tried several different formulations with the same active ingredients and again, some were helpful and some not.

It wasn't a question of merely changing supplements – buy one from me instead of the one you are already taking - some of the ones I was using at the time were also not good for Fiona. I was curious as to why and started to look more closely at the extra ingredients in the supplements. The common denominator seemed to be magnesium stearate.

I tested Fiona with magnesium stearate on its own, and it was affecting her. We were able to work around this with choices that didn't include it. I now test magnesium stearate with many clients like Fiona, and they do often react to it. The question I would like to be able to answer is, why?

The Science Behind Magnesium Stearate

Now here's the science: magnesium stearate is a synthetic ingredient manufactured by putting stearic acid and magnesium ions together. Stearic acid exists in nature in meat fat and plant oils such as canola, cottonseed and palm oils. Some of the stearates may come from bovine sources, but most come from vegetable sources (usually noted as vegetable stearate on the containers).

Cottonseed oil is part of the waste by-product of cottonseed processing. The vegetable stearate comes from hydrogenating cottonseed oil and canola oil at very high temperatures. Hydrogenated gas mixes with the oil under high pressure in the presence of a metal catalyst for a few hours. It converts the liquid oil into a solid fat that's known as a trans-fat.

There are acknowledged health risks of trans-fats and hydrogenated oils [243] [244]. Both cottonseed and canola are genetically modified crops sprayed with pesticides. The stearic acid used in excipients is purified – some would say this is a good thing, but it also means it's less like its natural state.

95

So, where is the research, I hear you cry! I asked the same question. I found a great deal of anecdotal evidence from health lobbyists to say that magnesium stearate was a bad thing, but this just wasn't backed up by creditable research. One could say that the available evidence was 'biased' because it was from health bloggers, organic farmers and the like. A lot of it referred to two research studies but, when I read these, the detail didn't support the headlines. I then looked at what the research *did* say.

There are a great many studies about magnesium stearate, but none of them evaluates the long-term effect on health. They're either looking at how to make it flow through machines better or looking at the mixture of magnesium stearate with active ingredients to achieve the best distribution through the tablet.

Some of the studies look at the effects of a drug that happens to use magnesium stearate as the inactive filler. There are studies on the best way of combining magnesium stearate with the active material in slow-release formulations to slow down the disintegration of the tablet to increase the length of time the drug will be active.

My conclusion from all this is that I know from my kinesiology testing that magnesium stearate can be problematic for *some* people. I found only one study concerning an allergic effect for one person [245]. There is no other research to explain why it could be problematic, and there is no research to dispute it either.

It's less of a problem in nutritional supplements as it's possible to choose a different formulation without it. However, it's found in many tablet medications too, although not in liquid formulations.

Other Excipients in Medications

Although these names may not be familiar, I've included the food source as well. These are all present in tiny amounts but if you have an autoimmune disease and you are looking to 'clean up' your diet as much as you possibly can, then knowing these may help:

- Dextri-maltose - from barley malt;

- Dextrins – this is primarily corn and potato, but can also come from wheat, rice, or tapioca;

- Dextrans – from sugar;

- Dextrose – cornstarch;

- Dextrate - starch – variable source;

- Maltodextrin - corn, wheat, potato, or rice;

- Pregelatinised starch - corn, wheat, potato, or tapioca ;

- Sodium starch glycolate - commonly potato, but has other starch sources;

- Look out for any starches; they could be corn, potato, or tapioca. They could contain starch from wheat.

Wheat Starch in Medications

Some medications include wheat starch. Wheat starch is what is left when you remove the gluten and proteins from wheat. However, it's impossible to remove everything. There are still trace amounts of gluten left.

In 2014 the MHRA (Medicines and Healthcare Products Regulatory Agency) database found that in the UK there were just 20 medicinal products mentioning wheat starch as one of the excipients. Nineteen of these were tablets, and one was a topical ointment [246].

The good news is that people who have a gluten sensitivity won't have a problem with wheat starch. Coeliacs *shouldn't* have a problem with this, but it's a question of the total load. If you are eating lots of products that individually fall below the threshold for 'gluten-free' (but still contain a little), this may add up to be more of a problem. The advice on this from Coeliac UK is that you can sometimes use alternative medications, and anyone who has any concerns about this should discuss it with their doctor [247].

If you have issues with fillers in drugs and supplements, you need to be vigilant. When you get a prescription filled, check the brand name that you usually have is the same as the name on the new tablets and not a generic replacement, which could contain different fillers. If the pills look different, again, check the ingredients and ask your pharmacist.

Lactose in Medications

Many medications contain lactose – it's an inactive substance, but it's included to stabilise the active ingredients in the product [248]. Pharmaceutical grade lactose contains between 0.012% - 0.029% of milk protein. If you have a severe milk allergy, it pays to know about the content of your medication. Dry powder asthma inhalers could be a problem, although aerosol ones are fine. All antihistamine tablets contain lactose, but the syrups don't.

Nightshades

What are Nightshades?

Nightshades, or *Solanaceae*, are a family that includes thousands of species of flowering plants. Many nationalities around the world use nightshades in their cooking. The nightshades include:

> Aubergines (eggplants), bell peppers, *blueberries, cayenne pepper, chilli pepper, *goji berries, gooseberries, okra, paprika, potatoes and tomatoes.

*While these foods aren't nightshades, they contain similar chemicals. In theory, they could cause a similar reaction although I've not come across any research confirming this.

Black and white pepper, sweet potatoes and yams aren't part of the nightshade family so can be consumed safely.

Nightshade plants may all seem very different, but genetically they're similar. They contain substances called *glycoalkaloids*, which are poisonous. These protect the plants from predators in the wild. Considering the size of humans and the size of plant predators we shouldn't be affected by these toxins, but many people are highly sensitive to them.

When alkaloids are broken down your body stores the remaining substance (solanine from potatoes or tomatine from tomatoes), so although the plants aren't immediately toxic in the amounts usually eaten, stress results in toxin release. Stress could be events such as pregnancy, starvation or illness [249].

The level of toxins can accumulate over time. The peak solanine level occurs in the body after eight hours; glycoalkaloids can remain in the body for up to seventy-two hours after eating them [250] [251]. The individual amounts in each food may or may not be relatively small, but the accumulation over several days may be enough to cause symptoms in sensitive individuals.

The Science Behind Nightshades

How do glycoalkaloids kill pests? They bind to the cholesterol in the cell membranes of predators. The binding affects the membrane structure causing the cells to leak or burst open upon contact. These cells could be anywhere, including the gut (think intestinal permeability, again) and mitochondria. I've not mentioned mitochondria before. They're our 'powerhouses' that transform glucose and fat into energy.

Glycoalkaloids are also neurotoxins – this means they work in the same way as nerve gas. They block the enzyme that breaks down acetylcholine, a vital neurotransmitter that transmits signals around the body. The result is to overstimulate the predator's muscle cells, leading to paralysis, convulsions, respiratory arrest and ultimately death.

Symptoms of Nightshade Sensitivity

Symptoms of nightshade sensitivity include any of the following:

- Acid reflux from capsaicin (taken from chilli peppers) [252];

- Arthritis [253] [254];

- Autoimmunity or chronic conditions. This problem arises where the body gets confused about what is 'self' and what is 'non-self' and starts to attack its tissues. There are many autoimmune conditions that you may have heard of: arthritis, Hashimoto's thyroiditis, Graves' disease, Type 1 diabetes, Sjogren's syndrome, Lupus erythematosus, and there are many more conditions that affect different parts of the body;

- When the intestinal barrier (your gut wall) is sound, the dangerous connection between genetic predisposition and environmental trigger can't occur. Food protein particles stay where they belong (inside the gut), and your body responds to them appropriately without setting off the more extensive immune system [255]. Some autoimmune diseases significantly improve by paying close attention to gut function in this way;

- Diarrhoea, heartburn, or Itching [256];

- Irritable bowels. Solanine and chaconine, which are naturally present in potatoes, may disrupt the gut barrier. These toxins are a critical factor in the development of inflammatory bowel disease. Interestingly, irritable bowel disease is most prevalent in countries where fried potato consumption is highest [257];

- Leaky Gut. Evidence shows that paprika and cayenne pepper break the bonds between cells in the gut [258] (see separate section on 'Leaky Gut');

- Mouth swelling (rare, but serious);

- Nerve problems such as nightmares, headaches, dizziness, and paralysis in extreme cases;

- Rheumatoid arthritis and swelling in the joints is a clinical manifestation of synovitis (inflammation of the membrane between joints that have cavities, like the knees, hips, wrists, shoulders, and ankles). Usually, the synovial membrane is very thin, but in synovitis it becomes thickened and swollen, causing pain [259];

- Trouble breathing (rare, but serious).

The Nightshades: Potatoes

Potatoes originated in the Andean mountains of South America. Spanish sailors brought them from there to Europe around 1500. The sailors used them to prevent scurvy (potatoes are high in vitamin C). They weren't widely used though, as people feared their botanical connection with nightshades: people already knew that some nightshades were poisonous. Between 1748 and 1772, the following edict was law in France:

> *"In view of the fact that the potato is a pernicious substance whose use can cause leprosy, it is hereby forbidden, under pain of fine, to cultivate it" [260].*

In the eighteenth century, the potato's popularity changed when a French pharmacist, Antoine Parmentier, engineered demand by creating a scheme whereby peasants could 'steal' potatoes from the King's 'guarded' gardens. He's also responsible for 'mashed potato', which made the potato into a different product unrecognisable from its original form and therefore more acceptable.

There are now over 4,000 edible varieties of potato. The Andes of South America grows most of them [261]. In the UK, there are 17 varieties of edible potatoes available in the shops, although you may find more in farmers' markets [262] [263].

The Health Benefits of Potatoes

Potatoes have many health benefits, including something called resistant starch - this means starch that isn't broken down in the digestive system. It's food for our friendly bacteria [264] and it protects the colon. Potatoes also have many antioxidants.

The Nutritional Profile of Potatoes

Potatoes contain excellent levels of copper, manganese, phosphorous, potassium, vitamins B3, B5, B6 and C, and more potassium than a banana.

Potatoes Under Stress

You probably never gave a second thought to what the humble potato could do *for* you, or do *to* you. Potatoes are safe to eat when the tubers are healthy, but they can bite back when they're stressed. They contain several toxins, including the glycoalkaloids found in the nightshade family in general, and putting the plant under stress during the growing process or after harvest will elevate the level of toxic chemicals.

Stress to plants is a real concept that causes changes in the levels of their compounds. Green patches (caused by chlorophyll when the tubers have been exposed to light, when they should be in the dark, buried in the ground) reveal stress in the potato. Blight has a similar effect. The potato increases chemicals called alpha-chaconine and alpha-solanine to fight off blight. These chemicals have antifungal properties. Potatoes are also stressed when the development of eyes shows the tuber is about to sprout.

A bitter taste is a warning sign that alkaloids are high. The most significant concentration of glycoalkaloids and other toxins is found just under the skin. Peel this away, and you remove a considerable amount of the poison. Frying potatoes makes the problem worse as this concentrates the glycoalkaloids and can result in digestive problems such as IBS and inflammation [257] [265].

We often think that food poisoning must come from a bug; we rarely, if ever, think of the potato that was on our plate! There have been numerous cases of food poisoning from toxic potatoes, possibly caused by any of the circumstances above, even after eating just small amounts. The symptoms of this are acute gastrointestinal upset with diarrhoea, vomiting and severe abdominal pain. Occasionally there have been reports of more severe neurological symptoms such as apathy, drowsiness, vision disturbances, confusion, weakness and finally unconsciousness [251].

The Science Behind Glycoalkaloid Increase in Potatoes

The average glycoalkaloid content in the peel of a potato can vary from 3 mg to more than 100 mg/100g of the peel. For peeled potatoes, the average content ranges from 0.10 to 4.50 mg/100g. The differences are mainly due to storage conditions, mainly related to light and temperature. Although the glycoalkaloid content can increase in the dark, the rate of formation is only about 20% the rate of formation in light.

The rate of synthesis of glycoalkaloids at 24°C (75°F) is near twice the rate at 7°C (45°F). In a well-lit area, the solanine content increases dramatically after twenty-four hours. It doubles for potato storage at 7°C (45°F), it is four times greater for potatoes stored at 16 °C (60°F), and it is nine times greater for potatoes stored at 24°C (75°F) (reaching 180 mg/100g peel) [266].

Potato cultivars vary in the degree to which glycoalkaloids increase due to adverse lighting or temperature. The King Edward potato, commonly used in the UK, is subject to a high rate of change [267]. Anyone who is sensitive to nightshades may want to try different potato cultivars to see if this makes a difference to their symptoms.

Top Tips: if you are sensitive to potatoes, look out for products containing potato starch:
> medications, baking powder, mixed spice, shredded cheese, glue on the back of envelopes or elsewhere.

Potato flour is used as a substitute for gluten in processed gluten-free bread and in sauces and thickeners.

Potato Cross-Reactivity

There is a possible cross-reactivity with birch pollen, grass pollen and latex. Latex is a standard component of many medical supplies, including disposable gloves, dental dams, intravenous tubing, and bandages. Consumer goods such as condoms, balloons, baby's dummies (pacifiers), baby bottles and the elastic on underwear also contain latex.

The Nightshades: Tomatoes

In the late 1700s, many Europeans feared tomatoes. It wasn't because they were part of the nightshade family though. Tomatoes became known as 'poison apples' because wealthy Europeans who ate them became sick and died. The real culprits were their pewter plates, which were high in lead. Tomatoes are highly acidic and caused the lead to leach from the dishes. It resulted in lead poisoning, but no-one made the connection at the time [268].

The Health Benefits of Tomatoes

Tomatoes have a dual personality. Their association with the nightshade family could mean pain and inflammation in those who are sensitive and yet, at the same time, they're excellent antioxidants and anti-inflammatory agents. They support the cardiovascular system and help lower the risk of prostate and other cancers.

The antioxidant lycopene in tomatoes may help your skin recover better from sunburn, although the idea is to eat it rather than put tomato paste all over your skin. Tomatoes also contain lutein and zeaxanthin, which are essential for eye health [269] [270] [271] [272] [273].

The Nutritional Profile of Tomatoes

Tomatoes are rich in biotin, copper, molybdenum, potassium and vitamins C and K. They also contain choline, folate, iron, manganese, phosphorous, zinc, Vitamins A, B1, B3, B6 and E as well as a range of antioxidants.

The Tomato's Nightshade Qualities

The good news is that tomato glycoalkaloids are much less toxic than potato glycoalkaloids, but all the different types of tomato contain glycoalkaloids, whether they're red, yellow, green, or ripe. Tomatoes produce two glycoalkaloids: alpha-tomatine and dehydrotomatine. Alpha-tomatine is the primary source. As tomatoes ripen, the alpha-tomatine levels drop significantly. Artificially ripened tomatoes may contain higher amounts of alpha-tomatine than sun-ripened tomatoes.

Tomato Cross-Reactivity

Although nothing to do with nightshade sensitivity, tomatoes have a connection with Oral Allergy Syndrome (see relevant section).

The Nightshades: Aubergines (Eggplants)

The first cultivation of the aubergine was in the 5th century B.C. Despite its long history, the early varieties had a very bitter taste. People thought they caused insanity, leprosy and cancer. For centuries after their introduction, they were no more than unusual garden ornaments. In the 18th century, growers developed new varieties that didn't have the bitter taste and aubergines became popular. The top five aubergine-producing countries are China, India, Egypt, Turkey and Indonesia.

Keep aubergines in a cool place, not in the fridge. The temperature in the fridge is too low for aubergines; if you have to keep them in a fridge, wrap them in paper towels to absorb the moisture. The bitter taste of aubergines comes from phenolic acid, which is also responsible for the flesh turning brown when the plant is cut open. It remains perfectly edible in this condition, even though it may not look too good. Don't store cut aubergine, as it tends to rot very quickly.

The Health Benefits of Aubergines

Aubergines are rich in antioxidants, particularly nasunin. This antioxidant helps cells to receive and use nutrients from food. It prevents toxins from building up in the body and causing disease. Aubergines are also anti-viral, anti-microbial, and anti-carcinogenic (protective against cancer). They protect the heart and cholesterol from free-radical damage. Heating aubergines increases their antioxidant properties [274] [275] [276] [277].

The Nutritional Profile of Aubergines

Aubergines contain good levels of copper, fibre, folate, manganese, potassium, vitamins B1, B3, B6 and K.

The Aubergine's Nightshade Qualities

Aubergines (eggplants) produce two glycoalkaloids: alpha-solamargine and alpha-solasonine. Solamargine is more potent than solasonine. The seeds and the flesh contain these glycoalkaloids. There is very little toxin in the outer skin. They're much less potent than the glycoalkaloids in tomatoes, which in turn are much less potent than the glycoalkaloids in potatoes.

The Aubergine as an Allergen

Other aubergine allergies that aren't nightshade-related are more likely to occur in countries that use many aubergines in their cooking. A study in Asia identified five potential allergens that can result in an IgE immune reaction [278].

The Nightshades: Bell Peppers

Most bell peppers start off with a green colour and undergo colour changes gradually as they mature. Although some varieties will always be green, they can have a vast array of colours, from the red and yellow that we see most often to ivory, brown, lilac, purple and even a very dark shade that's almost black. The darker colours tend to take longer to mature so they can be more expensive. The variety of colours gives us an equal variety in the phytonutrients that they contain.

The Health Benefits of Bell Peppers

The ranking of the world's healthiest foods shows bell peppers score at number one for vitamin C content and number five for vitamin B6 [279]. They're also very rich in phytonutrients, which gives them an impressive list of health benefits: they can reduce the risk of heart disease, obesity and conditions of blood sugar regulation.

They're very supportive of eye health (notably macular degeneration), providing the lutein and zeaxanthin that are needed to protect the retina from oxygen-related damage. Recent developments have shown they can also play a part in reducing amyloid deposits in the brain, which can lead to neurodegenerative diseases [280].

The Nutritional Profile of Bell Peppers

Bell peppers have excellent quantities of vitamins A, B6 and C. They also contain folate, magnesium, manganese, molybdenum, phosphorous, potassium, vitamins B1, B2, B3, B5, E and K.

Should All Nightshades be Avoided?

Whether you should avoid nightshades depends on the severity of your symptoms. The issue with nightshades is the possible overload of the toxins in the body. Your sensitivity level could be anywhere on the scale from just potatoes to the whole nightshade family, including the spices (though this is unlikely). If you can identify a specific trigger then, of course, avoid it for a fixed time, but work on all the ideas in Part IV: Solutions to improve your general state of health as a priority.

Oats

Health Benefits of Oats

Oats are high in soluble and insoluble fibre. The insoluble fibre adds bulk to stools and makes them easier to move through the bowel. The benefits are that oats ease constipation and make stools more substantial in the case of diarrhoea. It's undoubtedly a question of: "not too slow, not too fast, just right". When transit time is optimal we experience the benefits of increased satiety – a feeling of comfortable fullness after eating that lasts for several hours without feeling the need to snack.

The combination of fibres in oats leads to a slow release of sugars from the carbohydrates. We use glucose from sugar to create energy. This slow release maintains a steady blood sugar level that gives us just what we need without a manic burst of energy followed by a sugar crash and the 'hangry's' (feeling hungry and angry at the same time) that can come from more processed cereals or snack bars.

This quality in oats is due to a unique carbohydrate called 'beta-glucan' and can be very beneficial for anyone, but especially those with type 2 diabetes, cardiovascular issues and high cholesterol [281] [282].

The Nutritional Profile of Oats

Oats are high in biotin, chromium, copper, magnesium, manganese, molybdenum, phosphorous, zinc, vitamin B1, protein and fibre.

Top Tip:

You can increase the health qualities of beta-glucan by soaking your oats overnight in the same nut milk that you use for preparation in the morning. Don't throw the liquid away in the morning; it contains useful nutrients. The soaking process starts the breakdown of the oats so that there's less work for your body to do.

If you are cooking the oats to make porridge, it will take less time. You can do this for both hot porridge or cold 'overnight oats' [283].

If you are observant, you noticed that I said: "nut milk" and not "dairy milk". See the section on dairy milk for the rationale.

Oats and the Connections to Gluten

Oats don't contain gluten. However, despite their many benefits, there are a few reasons why including oats in your diet may not be such a good idea if you are Coeliac:

- Oats can be contaminated with gluten when the grain is grown in the field: oats and wheat or barley are frequently grown as rotation crops;

- Oats can also be contaminated in the food processing factory or at any stage of transport from farm to plate;

- Oats labelled 'gluten-free' are grown away from wheat crops and processed in facilities that don't handle gluten. These shouldn't be contaminated.

Avenin Cross-Sensitivity with Gluten

Avenin is the name of the principal protein in oats. Its chemical structure is similar to gluten, and this is why your body can *sometimes* get confused between the two proteins. Gluten antibodies may react to the avenin.

Oral Allergy Syndrome (Also Known as Pollen-Food Allergy Syndrome)

Oral Allergy Syndrome is common amongst hay fever sufferers. The protein structures of the pollen produced by some grasses and trees are very similar to that of different fruits, vegetables, or nuts. When your immune system reacts to pollen, it can get confused by the similar food structures and mount a reaction to the foods (see below).

It's so named because the responses are related to the mouth, causing itching and swelling of the lips and tongue. This reaction occurs within minutes of contact.

While these collections of foods may appear entirely random at first glance, they're linked by their botanical plant families. The Umbelliferae family, for example, contains celery, carrot, coriander, dill, and parsley, as well as many others. All the plants within a botanical family have a similar chemical structure, and your immune system recognises that similarity and reacts accordingly.

Silver Birch Tree Pollen
Hay fever symptoms season: February – April

Any of these fruits could react with silver birch tree pollen:
>Apple, cherry, fig, kiwi, lychee, nectarine, pear, plum, peach, persimmon, prune and strawberry.

Any of these vegetables could react with silver birch tree pollen:
>Beans, carrot, celery, green pepper, onion, parsnip, peas, potato, spinach and tomato.

Any of these herbs and spices could react with silver birch tree pollen:
>Anise, basil, caraway, chicory, coriander, cumin, dill, fennel, marjoram, oregano, parsley, paprika, pepper, tarragon and thyme.

Any of these nuts and other foods could react with silver birch tree pollen:

Almonds, buckwheat, hazelnut, peanut and walnut.

Mugwort Pollen

Hay fever symptoms season: July-September

Any of these fruits could react with mugwort pollen:
> Apple, apricot, cherry, kiwi, nectarine, peach, pear, plum, prune and quince.

Any of these vegetables could react with mugwort pollen:
> Celery, carrot and potato.

Any of these herbs and spices could react with mugwort pollen:
> Anise, basil, caraway, coriander, dill, fennel, marjoram, mustard, oregano, paprika, pepper, tarragon and thyme.

Any of these nuts and other foods could react with mugwort pollen:
> Almonds, hazelnuts and walnuts.

Ragweed Pollen

(Ambrosia artemisiifolia). Hay fever symptoms season: mid-September – mid-October

Any of these fruits could react with ragweed pollen:
> Banana, cantaloupe melon, honeydew melon and watermelon.

Any of these vegetables could react with ragweed pollen:
> Courgette (zucchini) and cucumber.

Sunflower seeds could also react with ragweed pollen.

Sufferers don't react to these foods when cooked as cooking breaks down the allergen's protein structure.

Rice

Rice supplies as much as half of the daily calories for half of the world's population. It was first cultivated in China six thousand years ago, where it remained until Arab travellers took it to ancient Greece and India. It spread to other parts of the world, often in conjunction with conquest and colonisation. The Moors brought rice to Spain in the 8th century, and the Crusaders brought rice to France. It was transported to South America by the Spanish in the 17th century.

In Thailand, the translation of the word 'to eat' literally means 'to eat rice,' as the grain is so important. Thailand, Vietnam and China are the three most significant rice exporters.

The Nutritional Profile of Rice

Brown rice is rich in copper, magnesium, manganese, phosphorous, selenium and vitamin B3. It also contains some biotin, choline, folate, iron, potassium, vitamins B1, B2, B5, B6, E and K. It's a good source of soluble and insoluble fibre.

Brown rice is the most nutritionally dense form of rice (i.e. it has the most nutrients). The polishing process that converts brown rice into white rice destroys many nutrients:

- 67% of the vitamin B3

- 80% of the vitamin B1

- 90% of the vitamin B6

- half of the manganese

- half of the phosphorus

- 60% of the iron

- all the dietary fibre and essential fatty acids.

Milled and polished white rice must have added vitamins B1, B3 and iron [284].

Rice Allergy

Rice is known to be a low allergenic food in the west, but there have been cases of rice allergy reported in Japan since the 1990s. Symptoms include IgE-mediated allergic reactions such as rash, hives, facial swelling, Oral Allergy Syndrome, rhinoconjunctivitis (nasal congestion, runny nose, post-nasal drip, sneezing, red eyes, and itching of the nose or eyes), wheezing and anaphylaxis [285].

Rice toxicity

If rice isn't that big a problem, you may be wondering why I've included it in a book about allergies and intolerances. The problem is arsenic toxicity. Arsenic is naturally present in our environment, which means it gets into the water supply. Rice grows in water in paddy fields, and the grain sucks up whatever minerals are in the water – good or bad.

There seems to be a difference in the way arsenic is absorbed in an environment where the plant is always underwater, compared to plants that aren't constantly immersed in water: the profile of arsenic take-up in rice is significantly higher than in barley or wheat [286]. It isn't just a problem that relates to third world countries. A 2012 study in the US found samples of rice contaminated at twice the level recommended as safe by the World Health Organisation [287] [288] [289].

In 2015 (to apply from 2016) the European Commission introduced limits for arsenic in food and food products. All rice contains some level of arsenic. Those who eat rice several times a day, or babies and toddlers whose first solid meals are often rice-based, may have a higher risk of arsenic poisoning.

The latest research studies available (2017) show that heavy metals still contaminate some rice beyond the level set by the European Commission, particularly in countries such as Bangladesh, Korea and China [290]. In highly industrialised regions there is also toxicity from cadmium and lead.

"I've been eating a lot of rice for years, and I feel fine," you may say. Arsenic toxicity takes years to develop. It can result in a range of health conditions including Type 2 diabetes, heart disease, high blood pressure, blocked arteries and cancer. It can also affect brain function [291] [292] [293] [294] [295].

Top Tips to Manage Rice Toxicity

- The experts believe rice is safe if you eat two or three portions a week.

- In some cultures that use rice every day, they soak the rice overnight and discard the water. When treated in this way, it's quicker to cook and also removes some of the harmful arsenic.

- Make sure you wash the rice with plenty of clean water before cooking. Keep rinsing until the water runs clear. Rinsing in this way should remove between 10% to 57% of the arsenic.

- Use plenty of water when cooking and strain the excess away. Using just the right amount of water doesn't remove any arsenic [296] [297].

The Food Standards Agency recommends that babies or toddlers don't have rice 'milk' due to their lower body weight (any toxins would be proportionally higher) and the fact that it's less nutritionally dense than dairy milk or nut milk substitutes [298].

Salicylates

Salicylates are chemicals that occur naturally in many herbs, vegetables, fruits and nuts. They act like preservatives to prevent rot and disease and protect against harmful insects, bacteria and fungi. The most vulnerable plant parts - the leaves, bark, roots, skin and seeds - store these compounds.

Issues with salicylates are best described merely as a hypersensitivity with a wide range of symptoms [299]. Respiratory symptoms can result in anaphylaxis, but less severe reactions are more common. In some cases, IgE allergy tests have been positive, but there may be other mechanisms.

The most frequent symptoms reported are:

Chronic hives or facial swelling [300], but symptoms can also include atopic eczema, flushing, low blood pressure, abdominal pain, diarrhoea and asthmatic reactions and occasionally severe anaphylaxis [301].

Top Tips – if you are sensitive to salicylates, look out for the following foods:

Apple juice, asparagus, Benedictine liqueur, black pepper, cardamom pods, cherries, cider, cinnamon, coffee, cranberry juice, cumin, currants, curry powder, Drambuie liqueur, fenugreek and fizzy drinks.

Also look out for Gala melon and ginger, Granny Smith apples, honey, kiwi, liquorice, mint, mixed herbs, mustard, nectarines, nutmeg, orange juice, oregano, paprika, peaches, peppermint, pineapple juice, raisins, raspberries, raw tomatoes, rosemary, rum, sweet corn, strawberries, tea, tomato puree, thyme, turmeric, tomato ketchup, tomato juice, Worcestershire sauce and wine [302].

Cereals, meat, fish, and dairy products contain no, or negligible amounts of, salicylates.

The number of salicylates found in food can be highly variable [299], and this can make it hard to pinpoint a culprit. Eliminating salicylates from your diet and environment is very difficult and isn't recommended as a first step. A better approach to exclusion may be to use the FODMAPS diet and then review whether different exclusions are necessary.

A 2015 review concluded that it *could* be useful to eliminate food additives and chemicals (whether natural or otherwise) such as salicylates, amines or benzoates from the diet for a limited period, if the remaining diet was nutritionally diverse and foods were reintroduced later [299].

Top tips – if you are sensitive to salicylates, check your medications:

Hundreds of over-the-counter (OTC) medicines and numerous prescription drugs contain salicylates - this information will be on the drug label. Aspirin is salicylic acid, and more than 10,000 tons of aspirin are consumed in the US every year. The quantity of salicylates in regular aspirin is typically 325 mg. Extra-strength aspirin or arthritis pain relievers can contain 600–650 mg.

In comparison, the daily intake of salicylates from food is estimated to be 10–200 mg on average, so it's far more likely that salicylate-containing medications will cause reactions than foods [302] [303].

Cross-Reactivity of Salicylates

Salicylates have a very similar chemical structure to other preservatives and sulphites and are a significant component of many food colourings and flavourings. Any of these could result in a cross-reactivity reaction.

Peanuts (These are Top 14 Allergens)

Peanuts originated in South America. As early as 1500 B.C., the Incas of Peru used peanuts as sacrificial offerings, and they had an essential role in aiding the spirits of the dead – they were entombed with the mummies.

Peanuts grow underground, so they aren't part of the same botanical family as tree nuts. They're from the Legumes family.

The Nutritional Profile of Peanuts

Peanuts are high in biotin, copper, folate, manganese, molybdenum, phosphorous and vitamins B1, B3 and E.

Peanut Allergy

Sensitisation to peanuts results in a very severe allergy. A US population-based study showed symptoms of throat tightness (56%), laboured breathing (43%), and wheezing (36%). There was also swelling just under the skin (51%), hives (42%), vomiting (18%), diarrhoea (14%) and loss of consciousness (4%). These symptoms affected one organ system (skin, respiratory, or gastrointestinal) in 42% of cases, two organ systems in 38% of cases and all three organ systems in 20% of cases [304].

A similar population-based study in the UK revealed severe reactions with a hospitalisation rate of 7.4% [305].

Adults and children are affected at similar rates, and the condition is lifelong (although research is continuing into this). For someone with a peanut allergy, cross-reactivity to other legumes such as soy is very common and it's best to avoid other legumes altogether.

Top Tips: if you are sensitive to peanuts, look out for these foods -
Any food including the word peanut (- butter, boiled, crushed, flour, ground, hydrolysed, kernels, oil, paste, protein, sauce, or syrup). Artificial nuts, beer nuts, crushed nuts, earthnuts, groundnuts, mixed nuts, monkey nuts, nutmeat and nut pieces.

Top Tips: any of these products could contain peanuts -
Arachis or arachic oil, arachis hypogaea, artificial flavouring, baked goods, chilli, chocolate, crumb toppings, egg rolls, enchilada sauce, ethnic food (-African, Asian, Chinese, Indian, Indonesian, Mexican, Thai and Vietnamese).

Also look out for fried foods, flavouring, hydrolysed plant protein, hydrolysed vegetable protein, mole sauce (a Mexican sauce), mandelonas (peanuts soaked in almond flavouring), marzipan, natural flavour, nougat and peanut butter.

Sesame seeds (These are Top 14 Allergens)

Sesame seeds could be the oldest condiment known to man. Their oil is very resistant to rancidity and so is highly prized. "Open sesame" - the famous phrase from the Arabian Nights – possibly reflects a fascinating feature of the sesame seed pod: it bursts open when it reaches maturity. Depending on the variety, the seeds can be black, white, yellow or red [306].

Health Benefits of Sesame Seeds

Sesame seeds are rich in calcium, copper, manganese, magnesium, phosphorous, iron, zinc, molybdenum, selenium, vitamin B1 and fibre. Sesame seeds also contain sesamin and sesamolin. These have both been shown to lower cholesterol and prevent high blood pressure.

Sesame Seed Cross-Reactivity

Cross-reactivity: people with sesame seed allergy may react to nuts like peanuts, walnuts, cashews and hazelnuts.

Nuts and seeds are often mixed in processing or passed through shared machinery in factories. It's possible for an allergy to be caused by accidental contamination at any time between harvesting the seed and getting it to your table.

Top Tips: if you are sensitive to sesame seeds, look out for these foods - Sesame seeds, sesame oil, benne, benne seed, gingelly and gingelly oil.

Top Tips: any of these products may contain sesame seeds - Bread sprinkled with seeds, hummus, sesame oil and tahini.

Soya (This is a Top 14 Allergen)

Health Benefits of Soya

Soya has some unique compounds called defensins, glycinins, conglycinins and lunasin, which provide us with health benefits related to improved blood pressure regulation, better control of blood sugar levels and enhanced immune function. Soya also contains a weak form of oestrogen that may help women after the menopause when their oestrogen production has declined [307] [308] [309] [310].

The Nutritional Profile of Soya

Soya is rich in copper, magnesium, manganese, molybdenum, phosphorous, potassium, iron, omega-3 fats, fibre and vitamins B2 and K.

Soy Allergy

Allergy to soy is most often a transient childhood allergy that usually resolves by the age of three [305], but certainly by the age of 10 [311]. Symptoms can be wide-ranging but not as severe as those caused by peanuts (a related food in the legume family). They include:

Diarrhoea, rash or hives, itching in the mouth, nausea, stuffy or a runny nose, vomiting, wheezing or other asthma symptoms.

Top Tips: if you are sensitive to soy, look out for these foods -

Bean curd, edamame beans (whole, immature soybeans), miso pastes, textured soy protein, soy flour and tofu.

Top Tips: any of these products may contain soy -

Soya is a staple ingredient in oriental food. It's also used in desserts, fillers in processed meat like chicken nuggets, frozen meals, ice cream, meat products, mayonnaise, natural and artificial flavourings, sauces, vegetarian products, shoyu sauce, some cereals, some peanut butter, soy sauce, teriyaki sauce, vegetable broths and starches.

Soy lecithin is a food additive used as an emulsifier. It also improves shelf life and controls sugar crystallisation in chocolates. It reduces spattering while frying certain foods. Most people who are allergic to soy may tolerate soy lecithin [312] because soy lecithin typically doesn't contain enough of the soy protein responsible for allergic reactions.

What to look for on the label:

Bean curd, edamame, hydrolysed soy protein, kinaki or Kinnoko flour (roasted soybean flour), Kyodofu (freeze-dried tofu), natto, miso and okara (soy pulp). There may be any foods containing the word soy or soya (- albumin, beans, concentrate, curd, fibre, flour, formula, lecithin, milk, nuts, nut butter, oil, paste, protein, protein concentrate, protein isolate and sprouts).

Also look out for Supro (a type of soy protein), tamari, tempeh, textured soy flour (TSF) and textured soy protein (TSP). Textured vegetable protein (TVP), tofu, yakidofu (firm tofu lightly grilled or broiled on both sides), yuba (bean curd), vegetable starch and vegetable gum.

Soya Cross-Reactivity

Soya has the potential for cross-reactivity to peanuts, cow's milk and birch pollen, which may result in allergies.

Sulphur Dioxide - Sometimes Known as Sulphites (These are Top 14 Allergens)

Sulphites are preservatives added to food and drinks to extend their shelf life. They work by releasing sulphur dioxide, which can irritate the airways and the lungs, causing them to constrict. This reaction is a sensitivity rather than an allergy because there is no IgE-mediated antibody response. The symptoms are very similar to an allergic reaction. Discuss them with your doctor, who may want to test for an allergy by testing for antibodies. The signs are a cough, gastrointestinal symptoms, hives, a tight chest, and wheezing. Sulphites can make eczema worse.

Top Tips: If you are sensitive to sulphites, look out for these foods -
Beer, bottled lemon juice or lime juice, canned coconut milk, wine and cider, condiments (all types of bottled sauces), dehydrated, pre-cut, or peeled potatoes and dried fruit such as dried apricots, prunes or raisins.

Also look out for fresh or frozen prawns, grape juice, guacamole, maraschino cherries, pickled foods and vinegar. Check processed meat products, soft drinks and vegetable juices.

What to look for on the label:
Sulphur, sulphur dioxide, sulphite, sulphites, potassium bisulphite, metabisulphite, sodium bisulphite, dithionite, metabisulphite, sulphiting agents, sulphurous acid, E220 sulphur dioxide or E221 sodium sulphite.

Also look out for E222 sodium hydrogen sulphite, E223 sodium metabisulphite, E224 potassium metabisulphite, E226 calcium sulphite, E227 calcium hydrogen sulphite, E228 potassium hydrogen sulphite, E150b caustic sulphite caramel and E150d sulphite ammonia caramel.

Tree Nuts (These are Top 14 Allergens)

Biblical writings in the book of Genesis mentioned almonds and pistachios as "some of the land's best products," and the Romans gave sugared almonds as wedding gifts.   Nuts are highly valued as their unsaturated fatty acids, fibre and protein help to lower high cholesterol, reduce blood clots (which could lead to heart attacks) and improve the lining of our arteries. They also keep us full for longer and provide a good dose of Omega-3 fats. There's no doubt about it; nuts are good for us.

Studies have associated eating nuts with an impressive catalogue of disease reduction, including reduced levels of heart disease, gallstones, diabetes, hypertension, cancer and inflammation [313].

The Nutritional Profile of Tree Nuts

While each nut has a different combination of nutrients, this family of foods are an excellent source of beta-carotene, copper, folate, lutein, magnesium, phosphorus, potassium, selenium, vitamins E and K, zinc and zeaxanthin.

Tree Nut Allergies

It isn't clear what causes an allergy to nuts: it may relate to your mother's diet when you were in the womb or breast-fed, or it could reflect cross-reactivity with peanuts [314]. Adverse reactions to peanuts and tree nuts account for over 50% of all deaths resulting from food-related anaphylaxis.

A minimal amount of the allergen may cause a severe allergic reaction [315]. If you are unlucky, a one-off incident may not be an allergy at all and may relate to salmonella poisoning. Tree nuts can transmit salmonella, but a 2017 study looking at 3,656 samples of six different types of tree nut only found 32 contaminated samples (0.8%) [316].

Until recently a nut allergy meant complete avoidance for life. However, researchers know that young patients outgrow 20% of peanut allergies and 10% of tree nut allergies by achieving higher tolerance of the antigens. There may be a small relapse in the number of cases of peanut allergy [317]. The only reliable way to test this is with an oral food challenge under medical supervision, as scratch tests and IgE tests aren't always reliable enough.

Top Tips: if you are sensitive to tree nuts, look out for these foods -
> Almond, almond paste, brazil nut, cashew, hazelnut, lychee nut (sometimes found in Chinese restaurants), macadamia, nut meal, nutmeat, nut paste, nut pieces, pecan, pine nut, pistachio, pralines and walnut [318].

Top Tips: these products may contain tree nuts -
> Artificial flavouring, baked goods, BBQ sauce, chocolates, chocolate spread, and crackers. Also look out for desserts, gianduja (a creamy nut mixture found in chocolates), mandelonas (peanuts soaked in almond flavouring), marzipan, mortadella with pistachios (an Italian meat product), natural nut extract, nougat, natural flavour, nut butter, nut oil and nutella®.

Tyramine

Intolerance to tyramine is a food intolerance caused by the lack of an enzyme called monoamine oxidase. How could this affect you? Tyramine is an amino acid that helps regulate blood pressure. Experts have known since the 1950s that tyramine can be linked to migraines. Scientists invented the first ever type of anti-depressant medication at that time. Called 'monoamine oxidase inhibitors' (MAO), they increased the levels of some brain chemicals which are related to mood: noradrenaline (norepinephrine), serotonin and dopamine.

The release of these brain chemicals also gives you a burst of energy and elevates your blood pressure and heart rate. Soon after starting the medication some people started to notice that they got migraines and their blood pressure increased when they ate foods containing tyramine.

However, it was only in the late 1960s when a clear link was discovered. One researcher noted that some people with migraines who also had a deficiency of the monoamine oxidase enzyme had headaches after they ate foods containing tyramine. MAO inhibitors have been replaced by other drugs for use in depression because of the complications associated with foods and interactions with other drugs, although MAO inhibitors do still have other medical uses [319] [320].

It may take twenty-four hours before you notice any symptoms, so make use of the Food Allergen Identifier in Part V: Helpful Resources to help you track the connection between foods and symptoms.

The Science Behind Tyramine Intolerance

Tyrosine forms from the breakdown of proteins. In turn, it breaks down into tyramine. Proteins in foods such as aged cheese or meats are naturally converted into tyramine over time. Sluggish digestion increases the length of time that food is travelling through your gut and this allows more time for bacteria to convert tyrosine to tyramine.

Tyramine needs an enzyme called monoamine oxidase to break it down. Some people don't have enough of this enzyme and can't break down the tyramine. It travels to the brain, where it causes nerve cells to release high levels of noradrenaline (norepinephrine). There is subsequently an imbalance in chemicals in the brain that can result in the pain of a migraine [321].

Symptoms of tyramine intolerance can include localised swelling due to fluid retention, hives, migraines, wheezing and even asthma. Some researchers suggest that up to twenty percent of migraines relate to food intolerance or allergy. Tyramine intolerance is one of the most common toxic food responses.

Foods that are high in tyramine:
> Avocado, beer, broad beans, chocolate, fava beans, fermented cheeses, fermented sausage, miso soup, red wine, raspberries, sauerkraut, sour cream, soy sauce, pickled herring and yeast.

Tyramine Solutions

Work on speeding up your sluggish digestion by improving transit time through your bowels. Simple ways to do this are to:

- Increase the amount of fibre in your diet (more on this later);

- Make exercise a regular part of your daily routine. Activity increases the blood flow and range of movement through your abdomen, which assists your bowel function.

Include the following sulphur-containing foods in your diet to assist the breakdown of tyramine:

Broccoli, brussels sprouts, garlic and onion.

Yeast

Yeast is all around us. It's in the air and on our food. When the Romans made bread, they found that if the dough became dried out in the sun, they could revive it by adding sugar. What they had discovered was how to ferment yeast [322].

Yeast is a living fungus. There are over five hundred different species of yeast, and within each species, there are thousands of different strains. They don't all work in quite the same way - brewers will use brewer's yeast for their fermentation process, but bakers will use baker's yeast for theirs.

There is even a yeast that's known as 'the traveller's friend.' It's called Saccharomyces boulardii, and it's used as a probiotic supplement to protect travellers against acquiring diarrhoeal infections in hot and humid foreign countries (it can do this because it's sticky – this helps it to latch on to bugs like E. Coli and Salmonella and remove them from your system before they can do too much harm [323]). Yeast can even affect the way a beer smells, so a 'flavour wheel' of yeasts has been developed to ensure that brewers can achieve the desired smell [322].

The Nutritional Profile of Yeast

Yeast is an excellent source of folate, iron, phosphorous, potassium, selenium, zinc, and vitamin B1, B2, B3, B5 and B6 [324].

Moulds, fungi (mushrooms), blue cheeses or mouldy cheeses are all types of yeast. It's a very challenging food to avoid if you eat processed foods. Yeast converts sugar into carbon dioxide and alcohol during food preparation and processing. Adopting a low sugar diet may provide benefits by preventing the overgrowth of yeast cells within the digestive system. Don't be tempted to cut out foods that are high in natural sugar. Just cutting out processed foods will be sufficient.

Common Reactions to Yeast

A yeast allergy may result in abdominal swelling, breathing difficulties, dizziness and joint pain.

An intolerance is far more likely and could cause any of the following symptoms:

Abdominal swelling, constipation, bladder infections, diarrhoea, difficulty in breathing, difficulty in concentrating, dizziness, fatigue, infertility, irritability, menstrual problems, mood swings, muscle and joint pain, osteoporosis, respiratory and ear problems and weakness.

The red, blotchy skin that sometimes develops after drinking alcohol relates to other problems, rather than yeast – it's far more likely to be connected to histamines or sulphites (alcohol uses sulphites as preservatives).

Top tips: if you are sensitive to yeast, look out for any of these foods –
Blue cheese or ripe cheese such as Camembert, Stilton, or Brie, dried fruits such as apricots, dates, figs, raisins, fish that's pickled, smoked, or dried, meat, mushrooms, peanuts or peanut products, pistachios, poultry, over-ripe fruit and truffles.

Top tips: these products may contain yeast –
Bread containing yeast (croissants, naan, pastries, pizza, pitta, most sourdough, and pumpernickel), Bovril, fruit juice in cartons,

hydrolysed yeast protein, hydrolysed vegetable protein and leavening. Also look out for marmite, stocks and gravies, sushi, tamari, vegemite, vinegar-containing foods such as grainy mustard, mayonnaise, pickles, relish, sauces such as chilli, horseradish, Worcestershire, and yeast extract.

If you are intolerant to yeast, you should avoid any products containing yeast for at least three months to see if this improves your symptoms.

How Does Stress Affect Food Sensitivities and Intolerances?

Our body has two states, which are opposites. We should switch between these two states many times every day. First, 'Fight or Flight' mode occurs when we are very alert and ready for action - just in case a sabre-toothed tiger might come around the corner. We can decide later as to whether that readiness will result in a fight or a run at the fastest pace possible!

When we are in this state, all our bodies' resources move towards supporting that alertness: our blood pressure increases ready to help the muscles in our legs and arms, our peripheral vision widens so that we can see every little detail of our surroundings, our heart rate increases to pump blood to our extremities. We stop digesting food. We could even lose control of our bladders and bowels – they're just not that important at that moment.

It seems that everything happens in slow motion. You can hear the slightest sound and detect the slightest movement. Your attention is at its peak level.

The second state is 'Rest and Digest'. It's the opposite of 'Fight or Flight'. Our blood pressure decreases. Our pupils narrow, and the pumping of our hearts slows down. The blood flows away from our muscles and into our digestive organs. As a result, they become more active. We could watch the world go by for some time and not be so aware of time or what is happening around us. Our brain activity seems to have slowed down a bit as well.

Think of lions in the wild. When they're hunting, their attention is 100% focused on their prey. They're ready to pounce at just the right time, and all their biological resources are tuned in on that moment. When they're in 'Rest and Digest' mode there is minimal movement on the outside – it's all happening inside.

The Science of Your Body's Response to Food

Complex neural and hormonal interactions manage the processes that control what happens to food in your gut. They include everything from the speed at which your food moves to how much of any given enzyme is made available to break it down, how much mucus to add along the way and a host of other factors that help or hinder digestion.

The nervous system influences the 'Fight or Flight' or 'Rest and Digest' situation through a major nerve called the vagus nerve. This nerve controls the calming influence on the heart, lungs and digestive tract [325].

Unfortunately, in our busy world, your body doesn't understand the difference between facing a sabre-toothed tiger and getting an important piece of work finished by today's deadline. The boss is leaning over your shoulder asking for progress, and that's enough to maintain that 'Fight or Flight' state all day long. Lunch-break? What is that? You can get through twenty emails while you are eating that prepacked sandwich. What flavour was it today? You didn't notice!

When we don't give ourselves the time to digest our food properly, we just don't absorb it. Our resources aren't in 'Rest and Digest' mode and digestive functions shut down – you won't get the stomach acid and digestive enzymes that you need, or the muscular action to churn the food in your stomach and then the peristalsis (squeezing motion) to move food through your intestines.

You already know that if you don't break down food into its chemical constituents, you can't absorb it. When you don't absorb nutrients from food, your bodily processes start to work sub-optimally, just as a high-performance car doesn't perform well with the wrong octane fuel.

When this happens day after day, is it any wonder that you start to get food sensitivities and intolerances?

Rewinding Stress and Restoring the Balance

Fortunately, we can resolve this situation. All we need to do is consciously to make space for that switch to 'Rest and Digest' mode: take your lunch away from your work environment and eat it 'consciously'. Make sure you include some fruit and vegetables in it. Go for a short walk outside to get some fresh air, if you can. Even a walk to the car park and back is better than nothing.

Play your favourite music to yourself at lunchtime. You could also try ten minutes' meditation with some suitable music through headphones. Make your journey home the time to switch off from work and allow yourself to turn your attention to your partner, family, or leisure activity when you get back. The more you practise these things, the more natural they'll become, and the less work stress will mount up and affect your health.

Can Food Intolerances Be Resolved?

Can food intolerances be resolved? To answer this question, we need to think about functional medicine triggers and mediators. What action or event *started the* reaction (the trigger) and what action or event is *sustaining* it (the mediator). If you don't make changes after reading this book, then your food intolerances and sensitivities will continue and possibly get worse, because the things that sustain the condition are still there.

If you consider the suggestions set out in Part IV: Solutions to improve your diet and your whole environment then your symptoms could start to disappear quite quickly. Changing your diet isn't a race. It must be done consciously at first; perhaps you'll need lists and to think about some planning. See Part V: Helpful Resources for tools to help with this.

How to Identify and Track your Progress in Dealing with Food Sensitivities

Write down your current symptoms, then give them a severity score before you take anything out of your diet as, once things start to improve, it's incredible how quickly you forget how debilitating those symptoms used to be. This forgetfulness is a deliberate mechanism that your body uses to protect you - if you *were* able to remember the exact pain, you wouldn't do it again (ladies, think of giving birth, and you'll know just what I mean!).

Also, write down any activity that you would like to do but can't do because your symptoms stop you. It might be something you used to enjoy, or it might be something new that you've never been able to do because your symptoms have been there longer. It could be anything from taking a lovely walk to playing with your grandchildren, socialising without the 'toilet location check' or flying model aeroplanes. Sometimes it feels hard to give up something you eat very regularly.

Debbie is a case in point. She said to me: "I've come to the end of my course of treatment with you and I don't feel any better at all." I asked her to rate her two top symptoms now, on a scale of one to ten where one is the best it can be, and ten is the worst it can be. Her top symptom was joint pain, and she scored this as two. Her second symptom was morning stiffness in the joints, and she scored that at two also.

I asked her when she last had the morning stiffness, but she couldn't remember. She wanted to keep the score at two because she knew she "did get it sometimes." We then looked at the scores for her symptoms when she first came to me. We recorded joint pain as ten, and we noted morning stiffness as eight. When I pointed these out to her, she said: "Oh yes, it was terrible then, wasn't it? I've improved a lot since then." She had simply forgotten.

Food Intolerance Cravings

A study of Canadian college students showed that 97% of women and 68% of men had cravings for certain foods [326]. How would you react if I told you that food cravings aren't your fault? Would you be surprised to know that that little voice in your head that told you to have another biscuit comes from your gut bacteria?

A 2014 research study [327] found that microbes make us crave foods that either support the microbes or crave foods that suppress competing microbes. They can also make us feel uneasy until we eat foods that they like. Unfortunately, this doesn't mean that you can relinquish all responsibility: these bugs aren't concerned about how their feeding behaviour affects you!

Cravings and Bacteria

When there is a high diversity of bacterial species in the gut, they expend some of their energy in competing with other species for more space. It means they have less energy available to influence your thoughts on food. Increased cravings and a more limited diet result in reduced bacterial diversity in the gut.

Families of microbes have different food preferences: Prevotella like carbohydrates, Bifidobacteria like fibre and Bacteroidetes prefer certain fats. There are other families of bacteria that produce a vital substance called butyrate, which is anti-inflammatory and anti-carcinogenic (anti-cancer causing). Roseburia and F. prausnitzii from these families like to eat carbohydrates and fibre, particularly inulin. Low-carbohydrate weight loss diets can reduce these butyrate-producing bacteria significantly, leaving you more likely to develop inflammatory illnesses.

Part III: Tests

Lab Tests

I've included a whole section on tests because this is such a controversial area. Some people think tests are always the place to start. Some people believe tests aren't reliable enough and are a waste of time and money. The truth is probably somewhere in between. There are a great many more tests than just the standard food intolerance test (remember the 'many causes' and 'many symptoms' problem).

The Range of Tests

It's useful to know which tests are available on the NHS and which tests you must do privately. Many of the private tests I discuss aren't available directly to the public – you need to arrange them through a suitably qualified practitioner.

Don't forget that you don't need a lab test for many issues. The practitioner's skill and knowledge will allow her to understand your medical history and interpret your food reactions. Work with your practitioner to find the best solution.

How Do I Get a Food Allergy Test?

See your doctor to arrange an allergy test through the NHS. Doctors aren't going to hand out EpiPens without a good reason. If you take a private test, they'll just send you for another one on the NHS, so there is no point.

The first test used for allergies is the skin-prick test. The nurse places a small amount of a liquid containing the suspected allergen on the back or forearm, which is then pricked with a small, sterile probe to allow the fluid to move into the skin. If the skin around the prick becomes itchy and red within fifteen to twenty minutes, that can indicate an allergy

Another possible lab test is a blood test to check for IgE antibodies. The nurse takes blood from a vein in your arm rather than a skin-prick, as more blood is required for this test due to the small number of these antibodies present, even if you do have an allergy. Each substance tested will require a separate test, so the lab needs sufficient blood to do this. It used to be called a RAST test (radioallergosorbent test), but most labs now use another method called IgE-specific immunoassay. Some doctors still call IgE allergy tests RAST even though this is a specific methodology and may not be the exact method that the testing lab is using [328].

If the blood test and skin prick test are inconclusive, the remaining test would be an oral food challenge. Here, you would eat increasing amounts of the suspected allergen to provoke a response. The test is carried out under medical supervision because if you *did* have an allergy, you could have a very rapid and severe reaction to the food and emergency medication may be necessary [329]

These tests may be useful for the doctor's initial diagnosis, but they can't be used to see if the person still has an allergy sometime later as IgE antibodies are long-lived – they could be in circulation months or years after the initial contact [330]. A new test would only show the original antibodies.

Allergy Tests outside of the NHS

Don't be tempted to find an allergy test yourself and then take it to your doctor. It has no validity within the NHS and will just cost you money unnecessarily. If your doctor thinks your symptoms aren't consistent with a food allergy, then it may be worth exploring food intolerances and food sensitivities.

Testing and Coeliac Disease

The potential for Coeliac disease is something you should most definitely refer to your doctor. The first test that she would do would be a blood test to look for antibodies or a biopsy to look at the lining of the small intestine.

If you are Coeliac, there is no point doing the medical tests again in the future. If you've been on a gluten-free diet for a while and then repeat the blood test, the test will very likely come back with no antibodies. It just means that your body is responding well to the gluten-free diet. It doesn't signify that you can reintroduce gluten. You'll never be able to do this as, if you do, gluten will start the same destructive process all over again [331].

Is it Essential to Get a Test for Food Intolerances or Sensitivities?

First, I want to clear up the definition of a 'food intolerance test'. Labs use this term to market directly to the public. What they mean is that they're testing for delayed immune reactions to food-producing IgG antibodies. Of course, we know that this is food sensitivity rather than intolerance, but I will continue calling it food intolerance (IgG), so you know what we are discussing.

If you had a food intolerance test (IgG) and you reacted to milk, for example, you would be responding to the *protein* in the milk, and it wouldn't be a test for lactose intolerance (because lactose is a sugar, not a protein). Again, this is where a practitioner can advise you on the right type of test to confirm or deny your suspicions.

It's essential to anything you do to ask yourself: "Why am I doing this?" You carry out a food intolerance test to identify problem foods more quickly. That's it. There is no other reason. Any test will cost some amount of money (it varies from one test to another) – you may deem that useful expenditure or you may decide you would prefer to do the elimination diet instead.

I saw one client, Gemma, with severe fibromyalgia who visited doctors and a range of different practitioners in her quest to get well again. Before seeing me, she tried eliminating lots of different foods in a somewhat random way but had been doing this for so long that she was missing all sorts of nutrients. It made things much more complicated to start with, as we had to unravel whether her symptoms were due to the original problem she was trying to fix or due to all the nutrient insufficiencies she had built up through having a very restricted diet for a long time.

When you eliminate foods from your diet, you *must* introduce substitutes so that you still have all the raw materials to function and build what your body needs. Adequate protein and minerals are very often missing when people take a DIY approach, and this is where a practitioner can help.

Many practitioners don't use food intolerance/sensitivity testing of any form and will base their judgement directly on the client's presentation: their medical history, the way they look, a standard physical examination and their symptoms. Many other practitioners will use different types of lab test such as a CDSA (comprehensive digestive stool analysis) to look at gut function, or breath tests that look for small intestinal bacterial overgrowth or H. Pylori – these tests are looking at a broader reason for dysfunction beyond just food sensitivities.

Some practitioners will use the 'elimination diet' as both a test and possible solution, by avoiding the top known problem-causing foods and then gradually reintroducing them to identify which one(s) is causing a problem.

Negative Feedback on Food Intolerance Tests

In my research for this book, I came across several very negative articles dismissing food intolerance tests. I felt dismayed at some of the wording used because, although what the reporters had written was correct, there was some information missing. I've included here my comments on some of the things you'll see elsewhere because I want you to have the best all-round knowledge with which to make decisions:

"Food intolerance tests don't identify allergies": this is correct. Food intolerance isn't an allergy – intolerance lab tests won't detect allergies because they aren't looking for them (remember the difference between IgE and IgG antibodies).

"A food intolerance isn't a disease or disorder": this is correct. If it were, it would fall within the remit of medicine, and your doctor would give you a drug for it. That doesn't mean it doesn't exist, or that it doesn't give you symptoms that affect your day-to-day life

"Where is the research?" Some people like to see many research studies to back anything they might do. I even came across one therapist who wouldn't recommend anything that she couldn't substantiate in a court of law.

Food intolerance testing (IgG) just gives you another tool with which to make decisions, but we need to get the right order of magnitude here: a food intolerance test isn't in the same league as a test to verify that a drug won't kill you or cause lifelong disability. The worst damage that it can cause you as the consumer is to make your finger bleed for a short while if you choose the finger-prick lab test route.

You can choose whether to act upon the subsequent report or not. If you take a new drug, one dose may be enough to cause severe harm or even kill you, and that's why those controlled studies are critical. Pharmaceutical companies need plenty of research studies for good reasons – not all drugs work initially, and no-one is prepared to take the risk without adequate backing. Someone must pay for research studies, and they're costly. You'll find a small number of research studies on food intolerances, but not vast quantities; in my view, you don't need them.

Your food intolerance symptoms have an impact on your day-to-day quality of life. You know when you don't feel well and how it affects you: you don't need a study to tell you that a test may be beneficial in isolating the culprit. If you don't have any symptoms, then don't do a test. On the other hand, if you feel it might be more beneficial to investigate further, some form of test (there are several mentioned below) is probably going to be very useful.

"It can't be true that food intolerance tests can show up anything from one food to hundreds of foods as problematic." This statement is false. The reaction to a food intolerance test is entirely individual, ranging from just a few intolerances to very many intolerances.

I tested one client, Patrick, using kinesiology. Patrick reacted to every single food in my test kit (one hundred foods). I'd never come across such a huge reaction before. It was so unusual that I re-tested several foods again, but the result was the same. He had severe diarrhoea and had to wear incontinence pants as the only way of dealing with it. It had been happening for at least the last six months, and I recommended he go back to his doctor as soon as possible to get this checked out as something was very wrong.

The following week, perhaps not surprisingly, he ended up in hospital. The hospital found that his diabetes drug, Metformin, was the cause of his problems (gastrointestinal disturbance is a known side-effect, not for everyone but severe for some).

It took a six-week stay in the hospital to 'sort him out' and, once on different medication, his symptoms improved greatly. So yes, it *is* possible for some people to react to many foods – but the question that we must ask is, what is driving that? What are the triggers and mediators (anything that starts or sustains a condition or problem)? Then what can be done to resolve the issue? As I've said many times now, the answer isn't to avoid all those foods.

"Pharmaceutical drugs can't cause food intolerances because they're tested in randomised controlled trials." This statement is false. Anything that you put into your mouth and swallow will go through the same processes as any food inside your body. Fillers in pharmaceutical drugs can cause intolerances (*some* nutritional supplements use the same fillers).

The fillers are there to improve the flow of the product through the factory machinery, and they make the product cheaper to produce. They have no health benefit to the consumer and are considered inert. In some cases, they do cause problems, although probably not for everyone.

The researchers test the drug's efficacy in a narrow range of parameters, as a drug to deal with XYZ symptoms for disease ABC. Studies need to have a small range of parameters so that the variables are controlled, and they can compare 'doing XYZ' with 'not doing XYZ.' I test people's response to their medications in two ways: does it help and does it hinder. It could do both, as they may respond well to the active ingredient but badly to the filler.

It isn't my remit to recommend people come off medications. What I can do is acknowledge there's another stressor on the body and make sure they boost nutrients for liver clearance (detoxification) or for membrane health (for the gut lining) or bowel function (to resolve constipation or diarrhoea), for example. Certain foods may help, or it may be that a kinesiology technique will help energetically, emotionally, or structurally.

"Some food intolerance providers also recommend a range of vitamin and mineral supplements and dietary changes to accompany the test." This is true. If you discuss this together with your practitioner, after reviewing your case (medical history, symptoms, and physical exam), then this makes absolute sense. The food intolerance test (IgG) is just one diagnostic tool of many that a therapist could use.

A combined package of test-and-analysis services like this is costlier of course, as you are paying for the therapist's time and expertise on top of the test itself. However, this is where you'll get the most exceptional value. I don't support recommending supplements based on a food intolerance report (IgG) alone – the individual is the essential element in any recommendations.

"The presence of IgG antibodies signifies exposure to food, not allergy." This is correct. Only IgE antibodies indicate an allergy. IgG antibodies are a part of the immune system. Your immune system is more active when you have a greater amount of antibodies. There is some debate about whether increased IgG antibodies are a sign of tolerance rather than a problem.

A test will tell you many things: not just which specific foods, but also how many. Whether your system has developed Oral Tolerance or not, somehow those foods encountered your immune system and it's just as useful to know that your gut needs some work.

"Non-standardised and unproven procedures: The (Expert Panel) recommends not using any of the following non-standardised tests for the routine evaluation of IgE-mediated (food allergy) ... Applied Kinesiology." In my view, this is correct, even though food allergy can be found just as easily using a slightly different kinesiology test, but I recommend that food allergies be taken straight to the doctor. Statements like this can sometimes be confusing for the public because by implication this method of testing shouldn't be used at all, even though that isn't what it said.

I use the analogy that no matter how good your electrician is you wouldn't ask him to do your plumbing because his skills lie elsewhere. The same is true of doctors and medical researchers. They know an awful lot about drugs and diseases, and they're the first people I would go to if I had problems in that area. Most doctors say food intolerances don't even exist so I wouldn't ask them about intolerances.

Although the kinesiology methodology would detect an allergy, food allergies should be diagnosed by a medical doctor because they can be life-threatening. If someone suspects an allergy, he should ensure he has the correct treatment available from a doctor (such as an EpiPen).

Where to Get Food Intolerance Tests

Does the NHS Do Food Intolerance Testing?
The NHS doesn't offer food intolerance tests. Bear in mind the nature of our health services: they're there to deal with disease rather than improve your wellness. Food intolerances and sensitivities aren't diseases. As soon as you mention food intolerances, you are looking for something outside the NHS remit.

Are Food Intolerance Tests Accurate?
The accuracy figure I've seen mentioned in many places is 85%, but the most critical aspect for me is just that they aren't 100%. If they were 87% reliable rather than 85%, would that make a difference to you? They increase the level of information – but that shouldn't take away common sense and the knowledge and skill of the practitioner in interpreting them.

Positive Results to Foods You've Never Eaten
How can a blood test show you have an immune response to food you've never eaten? Does this mean the test is invalid? Not at all. You may remember the various sections where I've listed cross-reactive substances.

All foods may seem unique to you, with different shapes, colours, smells and tastes, but the lab test is picking up all those cross-reactivities we have seen in this book, where one food is biochemically similar to another.

Can Medications Affect Lab Test Results?

Yes, medications can affect lab test results. Medicines like steroids and immunosuppressants suppress the immune system. Antibodies are part of the immune system. Therefore the medication will suppress them too. This also includes steroid creams like hydrocortisone and daktacort. Even though hydrocortisone is available over the counter, it has a substantial effect on the body and is more easily absorbed if occluded - this means if it's covered up with clothes for example.

Combination creams like daktacort keep cortisol in the body for longer and can invalidate some lab tests. According to the lab, Genova Diagnostics, it can take between six months to a year for the effects of steroid creams to entirely leave the body. Antihistamines and antibiotics won't affect the tests.

If you've been avoiding a food for a long time, because you suspect it gives you problems, then you may not have sufficient antibodies to register a response in a lab test. Once your body produces IgG antibodies to a food half of those antibodies will die off after a few weeks. Of those that are left, half of those will die off in another few weeks.

Successive generations of antibodies are 'trained' to recognise the target food, recognition of the enemy isn't automatically passed down from one generation to the next.

Remember, your immune system is an army. If your army meets the enemy, they train more troops (antibodies), but if the army doesn't meet the enemy, they train fewer troops in the next generation and fewer again in succeeding generations.

Eventually, the response will be so low that it isn't detectable with a lab test. The lifespan of antibodies is one thing that varies between the different types: while IgE antibodies (the ones responsible for allergies) are long-lived, IgG antibodies (the ones for intolerances) are short-lived.

Why Do Different Testing Methods Sometimes Show Different Results?

Sometimes different labs will show mixed results because they may have slightly different ways of sampling the blood, or their red-amber-green traffic light system may have different threshold figures for the level that constitutes an intolerance.

There is no point in doing a test with one lab and then paying for another from a different lab to cross-refer the results. You aren't comparing results on the same basis. If doctors used different labs for their blood test results, they would have the same issues, but they stick to the same one.

If you are going to re-test it makes sense to stick to the same provider and same type of test that you used the first time so that you are comparing like with like. Bear in mind also that your body systems are never static. Everything is continually changing, so the number of antibodies varies just like anything else. Food sensitivity can resolve in as little as three months, so if you retest after three months, your report may look entirely different.

Why Do DNA Tests Sometimes Give Different Results from Other Tests for Lactase?

Tests just give you a way to answer some questions, but no one proof gives you *all* the answers to *all* the questions. To illustrate this, I want to share my daughter's case with you: my daughter did a DNA test because we suspected lactose intolerance, amongst other things. I was astonished that her DNA test said she was lactose-tolerant. How could this be?

She had eczema almost since birth. While that was mostly under control, she had regular flare-ups throughout her life whenever she had dairy. She was having symptoms of stomach cramps and diarrhoea very shortly after drinking milk. I tested her using kinesiology several times over the years, and she was always lactose-intolerant; she reacted less if she drank lactofree milk.

I've seen this happen with other clients where the genetic test (a DNA test) says someone is lactose-tolerant – in other words, they *can* produce the lactase enzyme, but their symptoms suggest otherwise, and different tests also say otherwise. They know within half an hour (or less) of drinking milk that they'll get abdominal cramps and diarrhoea. Does that mean one/all tests are unreliable? No. DNA (our genetics) is very much affected by our environment (this is called epigenetics).

Our bodies need the right fuel to produce all those biochemical reactions that make us living beings. If we don't supply the raw ingredients for that, something will go wrong. In the same way, you wouldn't expect a carpenter to make you a table if you gave him glue and nails but no wood! If your diet is low in protein, your body will be short of raw materials, and it won't be able to make everything you need. In this case, lactase may be one casualty.

There's another reason you may be lactose intolerant when your genes say otherwise. If you've any degree of gluten problem (Coeliac or sensitivity), your gut lining will be damaged if you aren't already on a gluten-free diet. The gut lining produces lactase, so when that lining is damaged, you can't create lactase and therefore won't be able to break down the lactose in milk.

In conclusion, both the DNA and intolerance tests are correct, even though they give you different information. It does mean there may be a different outcome though: if the DNA test said you were lactose *intolerant*, this would be for life. If the DNA test said you were lactose *tolerant,* but the other test said you weren't, lactose intolerance is occurring as a secondary feature of gut damage, and it can recover.

In my daughter's case, she gets itchy dermatitis within half an hour of eating gluten and gluten is the primary driver; the lactose intolerance is secondary (she's *cautious* about eating gluten, but occasionally she misses something).

Kinesiology tests can give you a different view of how food affects you through tests for 'hidden' and 'overload'. A 'hidden' problem is one that doesn't show on a general kinesiology test, and you must dig a little deeper to find it. Perhaps it's something that has only just started to affect you, and it doesn't yet cause noticeable symptoms. 'Overload' is as it sounds. You eat too much of that food. Ease back, and your symptoms will reduce.

The Pitfalls of Food Intolerance Tests (IgG)

In my opinion, DIY isn't enough. Your body is hugely complex and is always changing. The neurons in your brain must last a lifetime, but your gut cells renew themselves every four days. The cells in your skin live about two to three weeks while red blood cells last four months [332]. Our bodies are constantly repairing themselves (the primary function of sleep). Raw data needs context, and too often people treat an intolerance report (however derived) as a list of forbidden foods. Food sensitivities aren't allergies, and you shouldn't consider them as such. A skilled practitioner can help you make sense of the data

Food Intolerance Testing Through Kinesiology

Kinesiology is the perfect fusion of eastern and western philosophies. It originated in the 1960s with a curious chiropractor in America who was interested in TCM (Traditional Chinese medicine). In all traditions, many significant advances in medicine have come from someone saying, "I wonder if/what happens when I do this?"

He discovered that applying light pressure to specific muscles and evaluating the response could relate to imbalances in body organs and energetic meridians. Acupuncture uses these same meridians.

Body scans reveal them as superhighways of light. They're single-lane roads rather than dual carriageways, and, just like our road system, can be subject to delays and blockages and even 'contraflows' when the body's energy isn't in balance. This imbalance causes us to feel unwell.

I've heard many people dismiss the concept of energy in the body, just because it doesn't conform to the western medicine view of how the body works. I compare it to electricity - we can't see it, yet we are comfortable with the idea that it travels through wires in the walls of our houses. A skilled kinesiologist can feel your body's energy in a similar way to the way you might feel a static charge of electricity, but this skill only develops over years of training.

When a kinesiologist does a test, he or she will first test a muscle 'in the clear' to calibrate the response. 'In the clear' means without introducing anything that could be a stressor to the body's energy. As this is physical therapy, it helps the kinesiologist to get a view of how that person's muscles perform before testing begins.

They're then better placed to interpret the responses. If the client is 'in balance', their energy is flowing correctly around the meridians. The kinesiologist will use a technique to temporarily change the response of the muscle to make sure that it's working correctly. Muscle responses should be binary, either feeling as if the person could hold that position all day or feeling like quite hard work [333]. The kinesiologist will either then use some other techniques on the client to get them to a state where food testing can begin or will be able to carry on with food testing immediately.

The food test consists of introducing various foods 'into the circuit' (this is usually placed next to the jaw or sometimes on the stomach) and evaluating the difference in test response. If the food causes no stress to the client's energy, then there will be no difference from the baseline test response. If the stress is too much, then the muscle response will change in an obvious way, and both the client and kinesiologist should be able to feel this.

Scientific Studies that Support Kinesiology

The more logically-minded of you may say: "but where's the proof! Point me to a double-blind placebo-controlled trial:"

- A small study comparing kinesiology and serum immunoglobulin food testing showed: "Comparable results in seventeen subjects with hypersensitivity, identifying the same food issues [334]. Kinesiology found 21 positive tests. The serum tests used both a radioallergosorbent test (RAST) and immune complex test for IgE and IgG against all 21 of the foods that tested positive with applied kinesiology muscle screening procedures. These serum tests confirmed 19 of the 21 food allergies (90.5%) suspected based on the applied kinesiology screening procedures";

- A further study evaluated the consistency of muscle testing between different kinesiologists, the consistency of results obtained relating to food testing [335], and a comparison of the kinesiology results with a food elimination and reintroduction protocol;

- The conclusions were that muscle testing was reliable between testers. Volunteers were tested with either a placebo or a nutrient. There was a statistically significant change in the muscle tone of the group given the nutrient measured approximately ten seconds after ingestion (p <.05), compared to the placebo group;

- A 15% decrease in muscle tone of the pectoralis major clavicular muscle was used as the criterion for detecting allergy. The muscle testing method was then compared to results obtained by a fast with the progressive reintroduction of foods. Correlation between foods identified as provocative by muscle testing and by the fast was 0.81;

- Observation of clinical results obtained with muscle testing suggests the method has substantial clinical utility. In summary, kinesiology muscle testing may be statistically reliable and valid for the rapid assessment of nutrient imbalances and cerebral food allergies. The method is appealing because both the patient and professional immediately see the effect of the nutrient on the muscle tone."

Scientific Studies That Don't Support Kinesiology

While there are a few research studies that support kinesiology, there are many that don't. Energetic balance varies from one day to the next: we often say "I feel very energetic today" (or the opposite). Even if we found a group of people with the same energetic balance, emotional state, organ function and resilience on one day, it could be different on the next day and probably increasingly diverse as time passes.

A double-blind placebo-controlled trial tests a small number of parameters against a generally-similar population, but in kinesiology, any imbalance in the body could affect a test result. For example, I could test tomatoes on three people to see if tomatoes are a sensitivity (I could use any number of people, but for the illustration, I will use three). One person may also have H. Pylori; one person may have a structural issue with their spine; one person may have arthritis. Any or none of these could be more significant than a sensitivity to tomatoes and affect the results. I would not be comparing like with like

The more people I added, the more variations there would be and the less common ground there would be between all of them. They may all test quite differently. In a controlled scientific study, if they were all male aged between thirty-five and forty-five with a 'good' diet and not taking medication, this would be sufficient to carry out the test. A scientific study is narrowing down the possibilities to the smallest number so that they can be measured. A kinesiology test is looking at the whole person – the broadest measure that can be found. The two types of test are opposites, but each has its place.

The Advantages of Using Kinesiology for Food Testing

- Many foods can be tested quickly and accurately in a short time

- Both the client and the kinesiologist can feel the difference in the muscle response.

- The results are instant. There is no need to wait for anything else.

- Kinesiology can test both intolerances and sensitivities - it isn't limited to checking proteins or antibodies. For example, it can also be used to test for lactose, where the missing lactase enzyme causes the issue. In this case, your body finds it impossible to break down the food. That creates stress, and that can be detected.

- Kinesiology can also test for 'overload' or 'hidden', where either too much of a food is causing issues, or where the intolerance response is at a shallow level but still causes an energy imbalance.

- It doesn't require any blood or lab work, so it's relatively cheap, requiring only the kinesiologist's time.

- The same foods can be retested later with no difficulties – there is no residual legacy of the original imbalance in the same way as there can be with antibody testing.

- Kinesiology testing can be as specific as the client chooses to make it – if they want to compare something that's homegrown from their garden with a shop-purchased variety, that's possible. If they want to find out whether food is the issue or anything added to the food (such as pesticides) is a problem, then that's possible. If they want to test whether eating something cooked or raw gives a different result, they can do so.

The Disadvantages of Using Kinesiology for Food Testing

- Tests shouldn't pre-empt the result. The client may inadvertently influence the outcome of the test by thinking about the foods. Sometimes the kinesiologist can feel this in the muscle response and will ask the client to think about the white ceiling or anything else to distract them.

- If some of the test results seem inconsistent, for example showing intolerance for cow's cheese but showing no intolerance for cow's milk. Cow's cheese is more fermented than milk, and the fermentation breaks down the proteins more. Some people who can't tolerate milk can tolerate cheese for this reason but not the other way around. The kinesiologist may retest some substances without telling the client what they're doing, just to re-check things like this.

- To reduce the possibility of accidental bias, Kinesiologists use plain vials that all look alike except for a name stamped on them. The client doesn't see the name, so they're less likely to influence the test.

- The kinesiologist may inadvertently influence the result of the test with a concept known as 'intention'. For example, if the kinesiologist knows the client's symptoms are consistent with gluten intolerance they may influence the test so that intolerance shows. Kinesiologists should always do a test with an open mind, thinking: "I wonder what happens when I test this?" Also, when I'm carrying out a food intolerance test with a new client, I do the test first when I've little or no knowledge of the client and *then* ask about their symptoms and history after the test so that I'm not biased. I just do the test, note the responses, and ask lots of questions afterwards to help me interpret what has just happened in the test.

- It's possible for food to cause an energetic short-circuit like blowing a fuse, with the result that any subsequent food tested will seem okay. It's just because no other response is now possible and all subsequent testing is 'stuck' in that response.

It makes sense for the kinesiologist to explain the testing process to the client at the start so that the client can appreciate the differences that the kinesiologist is measuring and feel included as a vital part of the whole process, rather than just having something done to his body with no understanding.

If the client doesn't understand the process, he can come away thinking it was all nonsense. Everyone forms opinions, every day, about many important and many trivial things. If you don't give the client information, they'll still form an opinion about the session, so better that they do this from a position of knowledge and understanding.

Food Intolerance Testing Through an Elimination Diet

In functional medicine, an elimination diet is known as 'the gold standard' because it's the most accurate and reliable way of identifying food intolerances. It isn't a test that gives you an instant result in the same way as IgE or IgG antibodies or kinesiology. It takes time and involves a measured approach to excluding the top known allergens and then gradually reintroducing them individually to see if they cause symptoms again. This approach is very useful where conventional medicine has failed to resolve symptoms.

Advantages of the Elimination Diet

- Whether the issue is a food allergy, food intolerance or food sensitivity, food is affecting you! The elimination diet helps to pinpoint what that food could be.

- Sometimes people don't realise just how awful they feel on a day-to-day basis until they stop eating the trigger food and feel better.

- There's a strong emphasis on a well-balanced and extensive diet, including foods from all the food groups. You don't have to work it out as it's all done for you.

- You aren't eliminating absolutely everything that might otherwise show up in a food intolerance test (IgG), but only the *most common* allergens from eleven foods or food groups. It does give your body the quickest opportunity to heal while lightening the load on your immune system. It will be a helpful start for many people and may be sufficient to uncover the problem.

- A phased reintroduction of the excluded foods also gives you the opportunity to assess how each food interacts with your body individually (see the Food Reintroduction Symptom Tracker under Part V: Helpful Resources. There is a downloadable copy of this resource on my website, www.oakmeadclinic.co.uk/free-stuff/).

- The elimination diet reduces inflammation, repairs intestinal permeability, and reduces the toxic burden, all while allowing an individualised approach with no calorie restriction.

Disadvantages of the Elimination Diet

- If your food intolerance isn't in the most common allergens, you'll see no benefit, and it could take some time to discover that, as you are re-introducing foods at the rate of only one food per four days.

What Foods Should You Exclude from the Elimination Diet?
The most likely contenders are:

- Beef;
- Coffee, tea, and chocolate;
- Corn;
- Dairy;
- Eggs;

- Gluten;
- Pork;
- Processed Meats;
- Shellfish;
- Soy.

What Foods Should You Include in the Elimination Diet?

- Fruits;
- Healthy oils;
- Lean meats;
- Legumes;

- Non-gluten whole grains;
- Nuts;
- Seeds;
- Vegetables.

Proteins help to stabilise your blood sugar so that you don't get 'the munchies' when you feel the need to dive for a snack. Good quality oils also help here. Legumes are a perfect combination of protein and complex carbohydrates – have at least one daily serving of legumes. It can take the form of soup, beans, a dip or hummus. It keeps you full and your energy supplying what you need.

It's a shock for many of my clients when we come to talk about vegetables, and I tell them the quantity they need. I'm not talking about five-a-day. I'm asking them to eat a rainbow of colours *every* day and aim for at least ten portions. Yes, ten. That isn't a misprint!

Let me clarify the size of a portion – your portion size should cover the palm of your hand (a larger person will have a larger portion size; a smaller person will have a smaller portion size). You might have two portions of peas as one serving on your plate, and that's ok if you are still managing to get the rainbow of colours over the whole day. It's best to work up to this level.

Suddenly eating a lot more vegetables could make changes to your bowel habits that don't fit your current view of 'normal' (because your view of 'normal' is just how it is for you), so increasing more gradually makes it more achievable. Include green vegetables. Cabbage is very helpful for an elimination diet, as the green vegetables help heal the gut.

See the earlier sections on histamines, nightshades, and salicylates. If any of these food families cause you problems, you would also exclude those from your elimination diet.

H. Pylori Breath Test

The breath test requires you to swallow a capsule containing urea. If H. Pylori is present the urea will be broken down and measured in your breath.

Advantages of the H. Pylori breath test

- It's available on the NHS, but only in cases of severe gastritis or suspected ulcer. Not all doctors will request it (if not, you can get it done privately)

- It's simple and easy to do

- It's very accurate.

Disadvantages of the H. Pylori test

- You must not take antibiotics or PPIs for a period before the test

- You must not smoke before the test.

According to the lab, Genova Diagnostics, breath tests are 90% accurate and can't distinguish between an active infection or a resolved infection.

Hydrogen Breath Test for Lactose Intolerance

Use this test for lactose intolerance. It shows the increases in hydrogen and methane that occur with bacterial fermentation of undigested lactose. It can be detected in the breath within one to two hours after exposure.

Advantages of the Hydrogen Breath Test for Lactose Intolerance

- It's very accurate

- It's simple and non-invasive

- Patients of all ages tolerate it well

- Many bowel symptoms are common to many causes, and this test establishes whether the problem is lactose [336] [337].

Disadvantages of the Hydrogen Breath Test for Lactose Intolerance

- False positive results may result due to the oral bacterial flora or if the patient didn't adhere to a low fibre diet the day before the test

- It isn't available on the NHS.

Comprehensive Digestive Stool Analysis (CDSA)

This test looks at overall gut health including digestion and absorption, inflammation, various markers that show how well the gut is functioning and the quantities and of 'good' and 'bad' bacteria. Parasitology may be added if required.

Advantages of the CDSA

- It's useful for a 'differential diagnosis': the same symptoms could point to several different problems. This test gives specific outputs to narrow that down, which, in turn, suggest possible recommendations for returning to health.

Disadvantages of the CDSA

- It isn't available on the NHS

- It's a stool test. Some people don't like to do these.

The Intestinal Permeability Test for Leaky Gut (Mannitol and Lactulose)

The intestinal permeability test is a urine test that measures the ability of two non-metabolized sugar molecules (mannitol and lactulose) to permeate the intestinal wall. The patient drinks a premeasured amount of lactulose and mannitol. The amount of the two sugars found in urine samples collected over the next six hours show the degree of intestinal permeability or malabsorption.

Advantages of the Intestinal Permeability Test

- People have used this lab test for over 40 years.

- It's simple and easy to do at home.

- It doesn't require blood.

Disadvantages of the Intestinal Permeability Test

- It isn't available on the NHS.

- Intestinal permeability can be affected by a wide range of factors which may not relate to the reason for performing the test (discussed in the section on Leaky Gut) [338] [339].

- If you have SIBO (small intestinal bacterial overgrowth) the test can cause some discomfort.

- Mannitol is a small molecule, lactulose a little bigger. Neither molecule is the size of a food antigen, and therefore the test may not be reflective of the immune response that would be caused by food.

The Zonulin Test

This test looks at the bonds between cells (the tight junctions). It's used to assess intestinal permeability or 'leaky gut'.

Advantages of the Zonulin Test

- Steroids don't affect this test.

Disadvantages of the Zonulin Test

- It's a blood draw.

- It isn't available on the NHS.

Part IV: Solutions

Healing Your Gut

I've talked a lot about the mechanisms for food allergies, sensitivities, and intolerances. I also want you to know that it's essential to look at the cause of the problem and then fix that. Avoiding the food will possibly give you relief from the symptoms (although there may be many foods causing the same symptoms) but if you don't deal with the cause, you'll find that food sensitivities multiply.

You might start off with just one or two sensitivities, but when you eat a lot of one food, and your diet gets increasingly restricted, you are very likely to develop a sensitivity to that one too.

Remember that too much of a good thing can be a bad thing – especially with foods like fruit. Limit these to just two pieces per day and stock up with vegetables.

There are so many ways to support your digestive system – and many of them don't require extensive thought or effort. The more you can incorporate into your daily routines, the better you'll feel!

Natural Enzymes in Foods

From my naturopathic nutrition training at CNM, the principle of "Food First" is always at the front of my mind. How can food help if you are short of enzymes? Luckily, some foods come with enzymes already built in to help us break down what we eat. Make sure you include these in your diet to give you a natural boost:

Amylase in Mango. Amylase is one of several enzymes that help to ripen mangoes. It breaks down starches into a two-sugar molecule (known as a disaccharide) called maltose.

Bromelain in Pineapple. This enzyme digests protein. You might recognise it if you've experienced a burning mouth feeling after eating too much pineapple – that's the enzyme. It's found primarily in the stem of the pineapple and its juice.

Honey Enzymes. These enzymes break down both protein and carbohydrates and include amylase (breaks down starches), sucrase (breaks down sucrose – another term for white sugar) and proteases (breaks down proteins).

Lipase and Protease. Food sources of both enzymes include legumes, all raw fruits and vegetables, sprouted seeds, raw nuts (not roasted, or heated in any other way) and whole grains. Cooking destroys enzymes, so it's a good idea to add some fresh fruit and raw nuts to your diet.

Papain in Papaya. This enzyme is a meat tenderiser.

Although avocados also contain enzymes, they also include other substances that may cause adverse symptoms in sensitive individuals (see avocados section) [340].

Increasing Nutrient Power and Reducing Lectins

All grains, nuts, seeds and legumes (beans) have natural protection - they don't want predators to eat them! If you are sensitive to lectins, poisons in lectins can irritate the gut lining and prevent absorption of some useful minerals. You can remove them quickly by following these tips. What is more, these methods make them more digestible and increase the nutrient content as well [341]:

Soaking and Cooking beans: this is the simplest way of removing lectins. Soak the beans *overnight.* Throw away the water and rinse again. Add sodium bicarbonate (also called baking soda) to the soaking water each time you change the water to reduce the lectins further and remember to give them a good rinse before you cook.

Sprouting: this method has been made famous by cookery writers such as Hemsley + Hemsley. Simply soak any seeds, grains, nuts, or beans for twenty-four or forty-eight hours, pour the water away and put the wet food in a container in the dark for up to seven days until it begins to sprout.

You may already be aware that this makes beans safe to eat, but it also unlocks the goodness in grains, seeds and nuts too. A study looking at the vitamin C and E content of grains found that sprouting them increased the levels of these vitamins (and others). The dry grains had virtually none of these vitamins. The content increased considerably seven days later after soaking and sprouting [341].

Cooking Methods

Using the appropriate cooking method helps by enabling you to absorb more nutrients from your food:

- **Include some 'raw food'.** 'Raw food' is meant here in its foodie sense of any food that you can eat in its natural state without cooking. It doesn't mean a piece of uncooked food that usually you would always cook – like potatoes or meat. In this raw state there is no heat to destroy any of the vital nutrients, and if you have enough stomach acid and enzymes to break it down, you'll be getting as much nutrition as you can out of that food. Think of fruits and salad vegetables – if you aren't a fan, try chomping on a raw carrot or a juicy red or green pepper for a change.

- **Many foods do need heat to break down the proteins.** Here, I'm thinking of meat and legumes. Heat also destroys parts of the food that may be harmful.

- **Gentle cooking is best.** By this I mean: use as little liquid, heat, and time as possible. I still have vivid memories from my childhood of boiled cabbage – the perfect example of how not to do it - cooked in a big pan of water on high heat for hours until it was transparent mush and utterly tasteless. Any vitamins that were initially in the cabbage ended up in the water, only to be killed off by the heat and evaporation. The cooking water was of course then just thrown away. When food is cooked at a rolling boil the individual pieces of food bump into each other, causing bits to disintegrate into the water.

- With large portions of food, the outside can lose its nutrients while the inside is still hard, so it's best to cut the pieces into small, even sizes so that you can reduce the cooking time and just use a gentle simmer. The result will look and taste so much better!

- **Roast or Bake.** Add just a little fat to the food, so *most* minerals, vitamins and other nutrients remain intact. The same principles apply regarding cooking for the shortest length of time necessary, so potatoes and vegetables chopped into smaller chunks will cook more quickly and lose fewest nutrients.

- **Simmer or Poach.** It's a question of temperature. Simmering and poaching are much more gentle – suitable for eggs, fish and fruit. Use this for tougher cuts of meat, soups, and stews. The temperature doesn't rise above 180°. It still allows the flavours to mix but doesn't break up the food.

- **Fry.** Frying is a rapid method of cooking, with the added benefit that the right fats and oils will help your body to absorb essential vitamins from the food (notably fat-soluble vitamins A, D, E and K). You should eat the fat as well as the food cooked in it so that you don't lose out but, equally, use only as much fat as you need and no more. See later for a further discussion about fats and oils.

- **Steam-Fry.** Add equal quantities of water and fat to your pan at the start of cooking. The water keeps the food moist and keeps the temperature of the fat down a little. You can still achieve a beautiful just-crispy texture without over-doing it (in fact, it *is* quite hard to overdo it with this method). Make sure you eat all the combined cooking juices and cooking liquid as it all has nutrients.

- **Slow Cook.** Foods are cooked in a liquid over low heat for an extended period. Slow cooking is best for crockpot style cooking with the whole meal in one pot. A lot of minerals and vitamins will leach out into the water (and indeed you may want that if, for example, you are making a slow-cooked chicken stew or bone broth using the chicken carcass). Add a tablespoon of apple cider vinegar to slow-cooked chicken to enable the bones to release their goodness. Do make sure it's an organic chicken though, as otherwise, you may be releasing hormones and antibiotics as well. Then throw the bones away and top up with more vegetables in the last hour or so of cooking. Finally, eat the lot!

- **Microwave**. Microwaves heat the food from the inside, by making the molecules vibrate and spin. Water-based foods heat more evenly, but fat-based foods are sometimes not cooked very evenly. The age and type of microwave oven may also result in hot and cold spots where the food isn't cooked correctly, potentially leading to issues with pathogenic bacteria. Glass is the best container to use in a microwave, as the heat can melt plastic.

Drinking Enough of the Right Things

Don't take hydration for granted. Our bodies are made up of 60% water [342]. You might be saying: "but I'm well-hydrated, I drink lots of tea and coffee every day." My first question would be: "how much is a lot?" Often we think we drink more than we do, and we confuse signs of thirst with signs of hunger and go and have a snack instead.

There is some good news for caffeine drinkers: while many say that you should reduce tea and coffee because they're dehydrating, the available research doesn't back this up. There is plenty of research that suggests the opposite but the tea and coffee industries commissioned this, and there is the question of whether this is biased.

Anyone engaging in sport or is in a tropical climate where they sweat a lot should increase their fluid intake. My view is that variety is a good idea, so if you really can't do without your morning coffee or tea, then go ahead, enjoy it – but have some water later, and try some herbal teas. There are different nutrients in all these things.

The connection with food sensitivities and intolerances is that fluid helps to prevent constipation. If you are constipated, the toxins in the waste will be reabsorbed back into the body along with the water in the stools, resulting in toxicity symptoms of a headache, fatigue and possibly hormonal problems. If you are looking to do everything you can to minimise and heal your sensitivities then checking what you drink should be a part of that too.

Improving Bowel Habits

Bowel habits are a result of what you eat and vary enormously from stools that are almost liquid to small, very hard rabbit droppings, and from going to the toilet several times a day to only once every three weeks (though, hopefully, that one is an exception!).

There is a very informative chart called 'The Bristol Stool Chart' which therapists use as one of their diagnostic tools to find out what is going on inside your body. It ranges from number one (the rabbit droppings) to number seven (the liquid mush). A healthy body should be around number four on the chart (a smooth sausage that's well-formed and very easy to pass with no effort).

There is absolutely no point asking clients if their bowel habits are 'normal' because they all say "yes." It's normal for them, whatever it is. As part of the journey to better health, I ask clients to increase their daily vegetables. That influences bowel habits due to the extra fibre (soluble and insoluble) in the vegetables.

A client once called me wanting to know whether it was a problem that he was now going to the toilet comfortably with perfect stools twice a day, compared to once every three days before! Changing the number of vegetables in your diet has a positive effect on comfort, body toxicity and mood [343] [344].

How Fibre Helps

What does fibre do for us? Well, quite a lot actually:

- Soluble fibre attracts water and turns to gel during digestion (think of what happens when you add water to oats – the mixture goes soft and sticky). Soluble fibre slows absorption. It's a suitable binder for substances like sugar and cholesterol. It has benefits in helping to regulate blood sugar, and some types of soluble fibre may help lower risk of heart disease. You aren't only feeding yourself but feeding your population of friendly gut bacteria too (see more below).

- You can find soluble fibre in oat bran, barley, nuts, seeds, beans, lentils, peas, apples, blueberries and vegetables. Psyllium is a common fibre supplement that you can buy in health food shops that you can use to help regulate bowel movements.

- Insoluble fibre is the tough material found in stalks and the husks of nuts and seeds. It doesn't dissolve in water (think what happens if you add water to celery – not much changes). It adds bulk to the stool, which helps food pass more quickly through the stomach and intestines. It helps constipation by adding volume to the waste material. In turn, this helps avoid problems like haemorrhoids [345].

- You can find insoluble fibre in foods such as wheat bran, vegetables and whole grains.

How Healthy Fats Help

Fat has been the enemy for many years. Public health messages demonised fat as the absolute enemy regarding weight gain, high blood pressure and heart disease, spawning a food industry bonanza by creating low-fat and no-fat goods. Unfortunately, health has not improved. The truth is, we need fat.

Why?

- Half of our vitamins are fat-soluble. If we don't include fat in our diet, we can't absorb vitamins A, D, E and K from the food we eat.

- We think of our cells as the flat circles we used to see in biology books at school, but a better analogy would be to think of them as three-dimensional pompoms. All around the outside surface of the cell, there are fronds just like the fibres on a pompom, and these need to move to let the right substances in and out of the cells through purpose-built gateways. They're made half-and-half of fat and water-soluble substances. Reduce the fat in your diet, and you risk damaging your cells because the cell walls become less flexible. Then they can't function properly.

- Your brain contains 60% fat – this needs maintenance and repair, and the sheath around our nerves is made of myelin, which includes fat.

- Our bodies use fat for energy. Some good fats like butter and coconut oil can be broken down in the stomach, without additional enzymes, because they're short chains of molecules. From the stomach, they travel directly to the liver where they can be used to produce energy. This energy creation happens in a completely different way to the method used to create energy from carbohydrates.

- Fat makes steroid hormones. You might be familiar with some of the names: testosterone, progesterone, cortisol and growth hormone (there are several others too).

- Finally, to dispel some more myths: eating fat doesn't create fat in the body. As human beings, we are a big chemistry set, and just about everything that goes through our mouth is broken down and made into something else. 'Good' fat makes energy. 'Bad' fat is toxic and is stored away 'safely'. Carbohydrates are broken down into sugar, which is rocket fuel to the body. It can't be used for any other purpose but to provide fuel with which to make energy, so the *excess* sugar (now in the form of glucose) is converted into *fat*. When you look at that cream cake or pasty, it isn't the fat that causes issues when you eat it (excess weight, clogged arteries, heart disease and more) but the sugar. (Although 'bad' fats – hydrogenated fats and transfats – have other issues that mean they should still be avoided)

These reasons come into play when considering the state of health of your gut, which we know matters in food sensitivities.

Using the right fats for the proper purpose is beneficial for health. Fats and oils fall into three simple categories – those that can be used cold as a dressing or a drizzle, those that you should use for frying or heating, and those to avoid.

Oils and fats with a high smoke point: use these for high-temperature cooking, such as frying or roasting. The fat molecule doesn't change shape with heat, so it can subsequently be broken down properly in the body. These are:
>Avocado oil, butter, ghee, coconut oil, duck fat, lard.

Oils that would be damaged by heat and so are more suitable for drizzling or dressings:
>Macadamia oil, sesame oil and walnut oil.

Olive oil fits into either category. It starts to smoke at 320°C/465°F which makes it suitable for high-temperature use as well as dressings, and it's used all over the Mediterranean for every purpose.

Oils such as canola, corn oil, peanut, rapeseed, safflower or sunflower are best avoided because they're heavily processed and contain high levels of Omega 6 (Omega 6 is an inflammatory fatty acid). Processed foods often use these oils, so check labels carefully.

Phytonutrients

Phytonutrients are chemical compounds in plants that are responsible for making them look, taste, and smell the way they do. Fruit, vegetables, grains, legumes, nuts, seeds and even teas all contain phytonutrients. Each colour has different health properties, so eating all the colours of the rainbow in a day is the best way to make sure you are getting plenty of these valuable foods.

The average purchase of fruit and vegetables in 2015 was 3.9 servings per day. DEFRA (the Department for the Environment, Food, and Rural Affairs) estimates that we waste 22% of edible fruits and vegetables so that the actual amount consumed is even less than 3.9 servings per day [346]. Here are some more shocking statistics from 2015:

- Only 24% of men, 27% of women and 20% of children (aged five to fifteen years) consumed the recommended five portions of fruit and vegetables per day;

- 7.3% of adults and 5.9% of children included no fruit or vegetables in their diet;

- Those aged between 65 to 74 eat the most fruit and vegetables.

Eating fruit and vegetables is one of the easiest ways to improve your health from any condition. Some people might cite the cost as the reason for not eating more, but the price of illness is far higher than the cost of a few extra vegetables. We seem to have lost the understanding that food is our first medicine; all phytonutrients are anti-cancer agents, but the various colours have different health-giving properties. It's better to increase the vegetables rather than fruit, as fruit contains more sugar and this can ferment in the gut, causing symptoms of gas and bloating.

"We Eat with our Eyes"

Marco is a client of mine who came up with this phrase, "We eat with our eyes," and I had to include it in this book because it sums up the wonder of the colours in fruit and vegetables. Try it for yourself; compare a plate of food that's all the same colour with one that has a variety of colours and see which one is more appealing. Not only are those various colours appealing to our senses but they each have different nutrient properties:

Red Foods – are anti-inflammatory, they offer cell protection, and they support the production of DNA. They also contribute to immune, prostate and vascular health.

Orange Foods – are anti-inflammatory, they offer cell protection, and they support the production of DNA. They also contribute to reproductive health, reduced mortality, skin health and they're a good source of vitamin A.

Yellow Foods – are anti-inflammatory, they offer cell protection, and they're helpful for cognition, eye, heart, skin and vascular health.

Green Foods – are anti-inflammatory and are helpful for brain health. They offer cell protection and help hormone balance, and they're useful for skin, heart and liver health.

Blue, Purple, and Black Foods – are anti-inflammatory, offer cell protection, and they help cognition and the heart.

White, Tan, and Brown Foods – are antimicrobial, offer cell protection, maintain hormone balance, and are helpful for digestive, heart and liver health.

Eating a variety of foods will increase the range of essential vitamins and minerals in your diet and decrease the risk of developing an intolerance to any single food [347].

The phytonutrients found in fruit and vegetables can be powerful aids in achieving good health and consequently overcoming food-related issues. We know that, over time, the food industry has reduced the bitter tastes that signify the presence of phytonutrient compounds through selective breeding.

Our palate expects a sweeter taste. How many bitter, acrid, or astringent foods can you think of - and what is more, how many of those do you eat? [348] Our food should be the ultimate nourishment, but we have removed many of the things that would keep us in good health. You can do something about this for your health by incorporating more bitter and astringent foods in your diet.

Top Tips: these foods will provide more bitter and astringent elements in your diet:
> Aubergine (eggplant), brussels sprouts, citrus peel, cloves, coffee, courgette (zucchini), dark chocolate, dill, fenugreek, grapefruit, kale, olives, radicchio (a type of red lettuce), spinach and tea.

Top Tips: add any of these astringent foods to your diet:
> Apples, artichoke, asparagus, buckwheat, cauliflower, cranberries, beans, broccoli, lentils, peas, pears, quinoa, rye and turmeric.

How Do Gut Bacteria Help Food Intolerances?

You have around two kilos of bacteria in your gut. These number tens of trillions of microorganisms from more than a thousand-different species of known bacteria. Human beings have about one-third of gut bacteria in common, but the remaining two-thirds are different from one person to the next. Each person may have around 400 different bacterial strains. The individual makeup of your gut bacteria is unique [349].

Gut bacteria are essential to our health for many reasons: they help to digest some of the undigested carbohydrates after stomach acid and digestive enzymes have taken their turn. They produce some vitamin B and K, and they enhance the absorption of short-chain fatty acids and promote storage of fats.

They train the immune system to respond to pathogens appropriately, and they keep pathogenic microbes at bay by outcompeting them for nutrients and other resources. Until recently researchers thought that the role of bacteria was limited to helping digestion, but now we know that they also balance mood and anxiety by opening communication between the gut and the brain, via the Vagus Nerve. (Vagus is Latin for wandering, and indeed this nerve has offshoots that do wander all over the body.) This communication channel allows the gut bacteria to influence your brain chemistry to increase the 'feel-good' chemicals [350]. Having proper levels of friendly bacteria can also result in fewer diseases such as diabetes, obesity and some cancers. These are all excellent reasons to look after them!

It's essential to keep your gut bacteria in the right balance to be healthy. Good bacteria (called commensals) are supportive as you've already seen, but the bad ones don't help us at all, in fact, they're just in it for themselves. What is more, they change the environment in the gut and make it less hospitable for the commensals. The 'good' bacteria can't thrive or colonise, and they die off in increasing numbers. It leaves a vacant plot for more unfriendly bacteria to move in. As diversity *de*creases, illness *in*creases.

I find the concept of 'The root cause of illness' in all the therapies I use. The question is, what causes friendly bacteria to die off? What is the

167

trigger? Did *you* have a trigger when you first started noticing food issues?

Things that will harm our friendly bacteria are any of the following:

- Not eating enough fibre (both soluble and insoluble);

- Not including prebiotic and probiotic foods in your diet (see 'Feeding your Gut Bacteria', coming later);

- Eating a lot of fast food or processed food, which is lacking in nutrients and high in trans-fats (also called hydrogenated fats, these are oils that have hydrogen added to them to make them more solid. They're used widely in processed foods);

- Not eating many vegetables;

- Eating a diet that's high in sugar or high in unhealthy fats;

- Trauma (physical or emotional);

- Illness requiring antibiotics. Antibiotics will kill off *all* bacteria, good and bad;

- Not taking probiotics after a course of antibiotics;

- Illnesses requiring medications which are immune-suppressant, such as steroids;

- NSAIDs (non-steroidal anti-inflammatory drugs) change the composition and diversity of the gut [351] [352];

- Feeling highly stressed for sustained periods of time, where you think there is nothing you can do about your situation.

Please take a moment to think about any food intolerances or sensitivities that you might have (or suspect). Think about how long you've had that problem. If you can pin it down to a specific month and year, that's great. If not, can you give it an approximate period? That will be better than nothing.

Can you remember what was happening in your life around that time? Even with an allergy that has a strong genetic predisposition, the genetics alone aren't the cause - they're merely one part of the puzzle. Very often, clients will say, "I've never been well since…." That "never well since…" moment is usually the trigger. There is often a succession of other things that happen after the trigger that keep you feeling ill.

Take the case of Cathy. She's now retired and came to see me because she was having pains in her abdomen, loss of appetite and a feeling of being too full and bloated after she had eaten. She had previously seen her doctor and took PPIs for years (Proton pump inhibitors reduce the level of stomach acid). She finally came to see me because she thought working on her diet more specifically might eventually sort out the problem.

She had already taken herself off the medication. I documented her full medical history from when she was a child. She had been quite sickly with lots of antibiotics. She never ate vegetables so never gave her gut the opportunity to nourish its population of friendly bacteria. Her "never well since…" moment came when her parents divorced when she was a teenager, and she moved to a new town with her mum, losing contact with everyone she knew and everyone who supported her.

Cathy felt very stressed and out of control. Everything was happening to her, and there was nothing she could do about it. She started to notice more digestive symptoms at this time. She succumbed to depression in her twenties and took medication for several years. She lost her interest in food and just grabbed the quickest thing to hand. She was married and divorced within the space of a few years.

This client has had a full life with many more notable events since then. The scene was set early in life, followed by a traumatic event that marked the start of her symptoms (the 'trigger') and then many other events since that continued the problems and in fact, made them worse (the 'mediators').

169

Cathy had many issues with food, but after adopting my various solutions, as set out in this section, she now feels better than ever. Cathy no longer has to avoid food or make excuses when she eats out or goes to a friend's house. She can eat whatever she wants.

Feeding Your Gut Bacteria (Your Microbiome)

'Dysbiosis' occurs when your gut bacteria aren't in the right mix of 'friendly' bacteria to 'non-friendly' bacteria. It isn't a disease, and therefore your doctor won't be able to help you with it. There's no drug you should take to fix it.

Instead, modify your diet to include more of the foods that friendly bacteria love, and they'll reward you by multiplying and improving your health. Your 'microbiome' (your population of gut bacteria), can start to change in as little as three or four days [353] [354]. The populations will be entirely different depending on whether you are a meat eater or a plant-eater.

Dysbiosis can cause issues such as:
> Bloating, constipation, diarrhoea, fatigue, food poisoning, IBS, mood swings, poor digestion and thrush.

The following foods will all encourage the right bacteria:

- Pre-biotic foods that act as food for the bacteria – artichokes, asparagus, banana, garlic, leeks, oats and onions [355];

- Green tea promotes the growth of friendly bacteria;

- Eat plenty of fibre to ensure regular bowel movements. If food stays in the bowel too long, it can putrefy causing many toxins to be released. It increases levels of the wrong bacteria. Find fibre in whole grains such as oats and brown rice, beans, fruit, lentils and vegetables [356].

Nutritional Supplements

Can nutritional supplements help? Some of them can, and I must mention them. However, my first line of healing is *always* through food, and I've stressed this throughout this book. I often say: "We don't become ill because we didn't take a certain drug," and the same is true of supplements.

There are probably times when a supplement is just what's needed – either to add in something beneficial that the body doesn't make, and has a supportive effect, or to boost levels of something that the body *does* produce, but currently is making in insufficient quantities. The need for supplements is very individual.

While people don't end up in hospital after taking the wrong supplement as they can with drugs, every practitioner has a duty of care to ensure that a client is using the right supplements for their needs – and no more. If your supplements take up a whole cupboard, or you have a shopping bag full, you certainly need a review of what you are taking and why.

Supplements should be checked against medications to make sure they don't change the way any drugs are broken down (and therefore change their effectiveness). They should also be reviewed to ensure they aren't doing precisely the opposite (taking a stomach acid supplement at the same time as using a PPI, for example), and a supplement regime needs to have a definite end date – it shouldn't be something that goes on forever.

In addition to this, not all supplements are the same. Some are very keenly priced, which may mean the addition of cheaper fillers and excipients in their manufacture. They may not be useful for everyone and, in some cases, may cause you to feel worse (see the discussion on magnesium stearate).

Supplements come in different forms - tablets, powders, capsules, and liquids. Some types are better for specific uses than others. It's best to work with a practitioner who knows which supplements to use in which circumstances. In just the same way as drugs can interact with each other, supplements can do the same.

If you're using several supplements you'll need recommendations about the best time of day to take them; what is the right dose for you and how to build up to that therapeutic dose. A practitioner will give you the benefit of her knowledge of using supplements with many clients. It can save you money overall, as well as help you feel better faster.

Easy Swaps

Instead of Beef

Beef is an excellent source of protein, so you shouldn't just exclude it. If you do, always make sure you are replacing it with a range of protein-rich foods so that you increase the variety of nutrients in your diet.

Try any of these sources of protein:
> Broccoli, cannellini beans (great northern beans), chickpeas (garbanzo beans), edamame beans, eggs, kidney beans, lentils, nuts, quinoa, seeds, seitan, tempeh, and yoghurt.

Instead of Dairy

Goat and Sheep Milk: you may be able to tolerate milk from goats or sheep, plus related products (such as cream, butter, yoghurt, and cheese) – depending on your test results. When it comes to proteins in your body, size is important! These types of milk contain smaller proteins so may cause less reaction.

Soya Milk Products: cream, yoghurt, and cheese - soya milk has been a staple vegetarian ingredient for many years, there are several varieties. It's available sweetened and unsweetened, flavoured, and plain. Most types make tasty sauces and soups. Soya cream works as a pouring cream, but you can't whip it. Soya yoghurts are widely available. Soya cheese doesn't taste much like a dairy cheese; perhaps it's more of an acquired taste!

Dairy Milk Substitutes: coconut milk is an excellent milk to which very few people react. Southeast Asian cooking uses coconut milk extensively. Coconut cream is found in tins and as a solid block, which needs to be broken down with hot water.

Other plant-based milks include oat, almond, cashew, hazelnut, and soya milk. These are available as sweetened or unsweetened varieties. If you are concerned about missing some of the nutrients in dairy milk, you'll find fortified versions that have added vitamins and minerals. The fat content of nut milk is lower than dairy milk.

Rice milk isn't a good substitute (see section on Rice Toxicity). Hemp milk is also available. It's higher in omega-6 fatty acids than other plant milks and can adversely affect the ratio of Omega-3 to Omega-6 fats if you have too much of it, leading to an increased level of inflammation in the body. It's okay in moderation and with such a variety to choose from, why limit yourself to just one?

Coconut yoghurt and coconut cream are also available.

Alternatives to butter: first, check that you are intolerant to butter before you cut it out of your diet as this may not be necessary. Just because you have an issue with milk doesn't necessarily mean that butter will cause you a problem, because it has a minimal amount of whey protein in it and a tiny amount of lactose.

Ghee is 'clarified' butter, which means butter is heated and the white foam scooped off the top. The white foam is the whey protein, leaving just fat (no protein or lactose).

If you want spreadable butter, mix equal quantities of butter (dairy or goat's depending on what you can tolerate) and olive oil.

I don't recommend any form of margarine.

Is cheese essential to you? The first step is to see if you are intolerant to cow's cheese. Cheese is made from fermented milk – the fermentation breaks down the proteins so you may be able to tolerate a small amount. If you can't tolerate cow's cheese, you may be able to tolerate goat's cheese or sheep's cheese.

There are quite a variety of hard and soft cheeses available now, so you have plenty of choices. Do remember to check the labels though. Feta cheese, for example, should be made with goat's and sheep's milk but sometimes includes cow's milk as well to make it cheaper.

If you just want the taste of a cheesy topping, try nutritional yeast flakes. They're a vegan product readily available in supermarkets and health food shops. They're made from yeast with a tangy, cheesy, and nutty taste, like cheese but nothing to do with dairy. They make a tasty condiment to sprinkle onto risotto and chilli to good effect. They also work well in sauces.

Cashew Nuts: cashew nuts can be used to make a cream (it can be savoury or sweet and made to the consistency you need), ice cream or mayonnaise. Dairy-free mayonnaise is also readily available in the supermarket 'free from' section if you don't want to make your own.

Ice-Cream: there are dairy free alternatives made from soy or cashew.

Chocolate: there are dairy-free alternatives available in the supermarket 'free from' section or online for everyday bars or chocolate-covered goods; there are also products for special occasions such as Easter eggs or Christmas confectionery.

Replace 1 cup of **buttermilk** with:
1 cup soy milk + 1 tablespoon lemon juice or 1 tablespoon white vinegar (let stand until slightly thickened.)

Replace **dairy yoghurt** with an equal quantity of one of the following:

- Soy yoghurt or coconut yoghurt

- Soy sour cream

- Unsweetened applesauce

- Fruit Puree.

Instead of Eggs

Eggs are an excellent source of protein. Other options are meat, fish, poultry, legumes, fruits, vegetables and enriched grains.

In general, try any of these alternatives:

- Substitute each egg with a mixture of 1 tbs of water, 1 tbs of oil and 1 tsp of baking powder

- One packet of unflavoured gelatine dissolved in 2 tbs of warm water (ready to use as soon as it's mixed)

- One teaspoon of yeast dissolved in 1/4 cup of warm water

- 1 oz. mashed tofu plus 1/4 tsp baking powder

- There are also egg replacers found in health food stores, such as Ener-G foods egg replacer.

Egg has a multitude of uses, from a binder to a raising agent, an emulsifier to break up fats; it's also used to coat foods or thicken sauces.

Ideas for specific swaps:

- In custard - use 1 tbs cornflour (cornstarch) per egg.

- In batter or dough, add 1 extra tsp baking powder for each egg omitted. If you want the product to rise: use more baking powder. Otherwise, replace one egg with 1 tbs vegetable oil and 2 tbs water

- As a binder, use either 1 tbs of unflavoured gelatine, 1/2 mashed banana, 1/4 cup creamy mashed white potatoes, or applesauce.

Pure powdered lecithin can be used hold liquids and fats together. Lecithin is a type of fat most often derived from either eggs or soybeans. If the lecithin is relatively refined, there is little chance that it will contain any egg protein. Use with caution if your allergy is extreme [164].

Instead of Gluten

- Instead of pasta use rice, buckwheat, millet, or corn noodles (you could also use gluten-free pasta)

- Instead of semolina, use polenta

- Instead of bulgur wheat, use rice

- Instead of couscous, use quinoa

- Instead of wheat bran, use gluten-free oat bran

- Instead of bread, use gluten-free bread as a first step, but there are plenty of alternative recipes using sweet potato, flaxseed and other vegetable or grain bases

- Instead of wheat granola, use oat granola mix (gluten-free).

Instead of Nightshades

- Instead of white potatoes try sweet potatoes or cauliflower

- Instead of aubergine (eggplant) try mushroom

- Instead of bell peppers try celery, radish, or courgette (zucchini)

- Instead of tomatoes try beetroot (beets) or carrots.

- Instead of cayenne pepper or red pepper flakes, try ground black pepper, or white pepper.

Instead of Nuts

Replace tree nuts or peanuts with an equal amount of:

- Pumpkin seeds;

- Sunflower seeds.

Instead of Onion or Garlic

Asafoetida (Hing) powder is a low FODMAP alternative, available from health food stores or online. It's always blended with something else so always check what this is if you have any issues with gluten – it could be corn starch or wheat starch.

Instead of Yeast

Bread:

- Try unleavened foods such as Matzos or tortillas. Soda bread doesn't use yeast. There is also bread that uses a different raising agent, such as bicarbonate of soda or baking powder. Pancakes or crepes don't usually have yeast in them (but do check);

- Oatcakes or corn cakes;

- Nut butter excluding peanut and pistachio. Cashew or almond are good choices.

Part V: Helpful Resources

Vitamins, Minerals, and Other Nutrients

Make sure you are having a varied diet incorporating as many of the foods listed below as you can [357]. I've not included figures for how much of the nutrient is in any given food because individual quantities of vitamins, minerals and nutrients will vary depending on the growth conditions and country of origin.

Furthermore, what amount is a good quantity? It isn't the RDA stamped on bottles of supplements you see in the shops. The RDA only gives you a level to prevent disease; it doesn't give you the standard for optimum wellness. Wellness depends on the balance of all nutrients for the whole person – not an academic figure for an individual nutrient.

Some people will need more of some nutrients, and less of others and a practitioner will help you with this. The main thing here is just to be aware that to support a fully-functioning human being is a complicated business. The more variety you can have in your diet, the more likely you are to achieve that.

Vitamin A
Function: vision, growth, immunity, and reproduction.

Best sources: apricots, broccoli, butter, carrots, egg, kale, liver, parsley, romaine lettuce, spinach, sweet potatoes, and winter squash.

Vitamin B (B1, B2, B3, B5, B6, B12, Folate)
Function: energy production, immunity, nerve function, red blood cell formation (B12). Folate also reduces congenital disabilities.

Best sources: beans, broccoli, garlic, lentils, spinach, tahini, tomatoes, oats, and pork. B12 - liver, salmon, sardines, beef and lamb. (Note: All B vitamins are water-soluble – steam vegetables to preserve the nutrients).

Vitamin C
Function: antioxidant (protects against damage), collagen formation (provides structure and elasticity for skin and tendons) and helps iron absorption.

Best sources: bell pepper, broccoli, brussels sprouts, cauliflower, citrus fruits, parsley, romaine lettuce, strawberry, and tomato. (Note: vitamin C is water-soluble – eat raw or lightly steam to preserve the nutrients).

Vitamin D
Function: bone mineralisation, calcium absorption, and immune function.

Best sources: butter, eggs, liver, oily fish (salmon, sardines, mackerel) and sunshine.

Vitamin E
Function: antioxidant and supports immune function.

Best sources: almonds, bell peppers, blueberries, brussels sprouts, kale, kiwi, olives, sunflower seeds, peanuts, spinach, and papaya.

Vitamin K
Function: blood clotting and bone health.

Best sources: basil, broccoli, brussels sprouts, cabbage, kale, parsley, romaine lettuce and spinach.

Calcium
Function: bone and tooth health, heart rate regulation, muscle contraction and nerve signalling.

Best sources: basil, broccoli, cabbage, canned fish (those that include the edible bones), celery, cheese, cinnamon, dried fruit, kale, milk, nuts, rosemary, romaine lettuce, spinach, sesame seeds, and yoghurt. (Note: calcium is water soluble – ideally steam or boil vegetables in a little water, then use the water in soups, gravy, and sauces).

Iron
Function: enzyme and DNA formation, supports immune function, oxygen transport and red blood cell formation.

Best sources: basil, beans, beef, broccoli, cinnamon, green beans, kale, lentils, lamb, liver, mushrooms, nuts, olives, parsley, prawns, pumpkin, romaine lettuce, seeds, shitake mushrooms, spinach, tofu and turmeric.

Iodine
Function: supports cell metabolism, helps to create thyroid hormones.

Best sources: baked potato with the skin, cod, dried seaweed, marsh samphire (a salty sea vegetable), nori (sheets of seaweed used in sushi), and milk.

Magnesium
Function: energy production, supports the immune system, muscle relaxation and nerve signalling.

Best sources: almonds, artichokes, avocado, basil, banana, black beans, broccoli, cashew nuts, celery, chard, coriander and cucumber, dark chocolate, figs, flaxseed, goat's cheese, green beans, kale, pumpkin seeds, salmon, spinach, sunflower and sesame seeds, yoghurt or kefir.

Manganese
Function: forms connective tissue, bones, blood clotting factors and sex hormones. Supports fat and carbohydrate metabolism, calcium absorption, blood sugar regulation, brain and nerve function.

Best sources: black pepper, cinnamon, garlic, grapes, kale, pineapple, raspberries, romaine lettuce, spinach and turmeric.

Potassium
Function: fluid balance and hydration, important electrolyte, supports muscle contraction and nerve signalling.

Best sources: apricots, broccoli, banana, celery, cucumbers, pinto beans, potato, spinach, turmeric and winter squash.

Selenium

Function: antioxidant and supports thyroid metabolism.

Best sources: beef, brazil nuts, chicken, cod, halibut, lamb, oysters, salmon, sardines, scallops, seeds (chia, flax, pumpkin, sesame, sunflower), shrimp and turkey.

Tryptophan

Function: needed to produce serotonin, the 'feel good' hormone.

Best sources: asparagus, broccoli, cauliflower, chicken, cod, eggs, lamb, mustard seeds, prawns, sardines, salmon, scallops, spinach, tofu and turkey.

Zinc

Function: used for carbohydrate metabolism, supports cell division, immune function and wound healing.

Best sources: beef, brown rice, chicken, cocoa, pork, pumpkin seeds, oysters and whole wheat flour.

Choline

Function: vital for nerves and muscles to function correctly, also helps brain development and memory.

Best sources: beetroot, eggs, fish, liver, meat, peanuts, poultry, shellfish, spinach and whole grains.

Lutein and Zeaxanthin

Function: powerful antioxidants that build up in the retina of the eye to prevent cataracts and macular degeneration.

Best sources: broccoli, brussels sprouts, chicory, and courgette (zucchini), eggs, grapes, green or yellow vegetables, green leafy vegetables like kale and spinach, kiwi fruit, paprika, parsley, peas, radicchio (a type of red lettuce), red pepper, rocket (arugula) and swiss chard.

Food Allergen Identifier

If you suspect you have an allergy to a food but don't know what it is, use this identifier to capture all the information to take to your doctor. You'll need to write down everything that you eat and drink – including medications, supplements and all snacks. Use a new form for each day and capture the information for two weeks. Note: this form can be helpful to identify suspected *IgE allergies*, which have a rapid response time. Don't use it for *sensitivities* due to the difficulty of associating food with a symptom when there could potentially be a long-time delay between eating a food and symptoms appearing.

Name			Date	
Time	Food/drink	Quantity	Symptoms	Duration of Symptoms

Food Re-introduction Checklist

Reintroduce only one new food at a time. Eat it two to three times on the same day, then write down any reactions over the next four days. If you don't react, keep that food in your diet and continue with the next food for reintroduction. If you aren't sure whether you reacted, retest the same food again. If you need to write more, just copy the blank chart.

	Day 1	Day 2	Day 3	Day 4
Time				
Food				
Digestion/Bowel function				
Joint/Muscle Aches				
Energy level				
Sleep				
Kidney/bladder function				
Headache/Pressure				
Skin				
Nasal or chest congestion				
Other Symptoms				

A Guide to Eating Gluten-Free

	Gluten-free	Need to check	Not gluten-free
Grains and alternatives	Amaranth, buckwheat, chestnut, corn (maize), millet, polenta (cornmeal), quinoa, rice, sago, sorghum, soya, tapioca, teff		Barley, bulgur wheat, couscous, Dinkel, durum wheat, einkorn, emmer wheat, Khorasan wheat (commercially known as Kamut®), rye, semolina, spelt, triticale, wheat
Flours	All flours that are labelled gluten-free *(E.g., Dove's Farm gluten free),*		Flours made from wheat, rye or barley, e.g. plain flour, self-raising flour etc *May be able to tolerate spelt – wheat free but not g/free.*
Oats	Most people can eat oats, porridge, oatcakes, and oat-based products	Oat cereals that have a mix of grains *(UK oats can't be guaranteed g/free)*	Porridge oats, oat milk, oat-based snacks that aren't labelled g/free
Bread, cakes and biscuits	All products labelled gluten-free including biscuits, bread, cakes, crackers, muffins, pizza	Macaroons, meringues *(Mrs Crimbles are g/free. Supermarket brands aren't unless labelled 'free from')*	All biscuits, bread, cakes, chapattis, crackers, muffins, pastries and pizza bases made from wheat, spelt, rye or barley flour

	Gluten-free	Need to check	Not gluten-free
	bases, rolls, scones		
Breakfast cereals	All products labelled gluten-free including millet porridge, muesli, rice porridge, corn and rice-based cereals	Buckwheat, corn, millet and rice-based breakfast cereals and those that contain barley, malt extract	Muesli, wheat-based breakfast cereals
Pasta and noodles	All products labelled gluten-free including corn (maize) pasta, quinoa pasta, rice noodles, rice pasta		Canned, dried, and fresh wheat noodles and pasta, gnocchi
Meat and poultry	All fresh meats and poultry, cured pure meats, plain cooked meats, smoked meats (e.g. Black Farmer sausages)	Any meat or poultry marinated or in a sauce, burgers, meat pastes, pâtés, sausages	Meat and poultry cooked in batter or breadcrumbs, breaded ham, faggots, haggis, rissoles
Meatless alternatives	Plain tofu	Marinated tofu, soya mince, falafel, vegetable, and bean burgers	Quorn
Fish and shellfish	All dried, fresh, kippered, and	Fish pastes, fish pâtés, fish in sauce	Fish or shellfish in batter or

	Gluten-free	**Need to check**	**Not gluten-free**
	smoked fish, shellfish, fish canned in brine, oil, and water		breadcrumbs, fish cakes, fish fingers, taramasalata
Cheese and eggs	All cheese except some soft, spreadable cheese. All eggs	Some soft, spreadable cheeses	Scotch eggs
Milk and milk products	All milk (liquid and dried), all cream (single, double, whipping, clotted, soured and Crème Fraiche), buttermilk, plain fromage frais, plain yoghurt	Coffee and tea whiteners, fruit and flavoured yoghurt or fromage frais, soya desserts, rice milk, soya milk	Yoghurt with muesli or whole grains
Fats and oils	Butter, cooking oils, ghee, lard, margarine, reduced and low-fat spreads		Suet
Fruits and vegetables	All canned, dried, fresh, frozen, and juiced pure fruits and vegetables, pickled	Fruit pie fillings, processed vegetable products (such as	Vegetables and fruit in batter, breadcrumbs or dusted with flour

	Gluten-free	Need to check	Not gluten-free
	vegetables in vinegar	cauliflower cheese)	
Potatoes	All plain potatoes, baked, boiled, or mashed	Oven, deep fried, microwave and frozen chips, instant mash, potato waffles, ready to roast potatoes	Potatoes in batter, breadcrumbs or dusted with flour, potato croquettes
Nuts, seeds and pulses	Plain nuts and seeds, all pulses (peas, beans, lentils), tahini	Dry roasted nuts, pulses in flavoured sauce (such as baked beans), hummus	
Savoury snacks	Homemade popcorn, plain rice cakes	Flavoured popcorn, potato and vegetable crisps, flavoured rice cakes and rice crackers	Snacks made from wheat, rye or barley, pretzels, breadsticks
Preserves and spreads	Conserves, glucose syrup, golden syrup, honey, jam, marmalade, molasses, treacle, maple syrup	Lemon curd, mincemeat, peanut and other nut butter, yeast extract	
Soups, sauces, pickles and seasonings	All vinegar (including barley malt vinegar), garlic puree, ground	Blended seasonings, brown sauce, canned, packet or	Chinese soy sauce

	Gluten-free	Need to check	Not gluten-free
	pepper, individual herbs and spices, mint sauce, mixed herbs and spices, mustard powder, salt, tomato puree, Worcestershire sauce	fresh soups, chutney, curry powder, dressings, gravy granules, mayonnaise, mustard products (such as English mustard), packed and jarred sauces and mixes, pickles, salad cream, stock cubes, tamari (Japanese soy sauce), tomato sauce	
Confection'y and desserts	Gluten-free ice cream cones, jelly, Swedish glace, liquorice root, seaside rock	Chocolates, ice cream, mousses, sweets, tapioca pudding	Ice cream cones and wafers, liquorice sweets, puddings made using semolina or wheat flour
Drinks	Cocoa, coffee, fruit juice, ginger beer, squash, tea, water	Cloudy fizzy drinks, drinking chocolate	Barley waters and squash, malted milk drinks
Alcohol	Cider, gluten-free beers and lagers, liqueurs, port,		Ales, beers, lagers, stouts

	Gluten-free	Need to check	Not gluten-free
	sherry, spirits, wine		
Home baking	Arrowroot, artificial sweeteners, bicarbonate of soda, cornstarch (flour), cream of tartar, food colouring, gelatine, icing sugar, potato starch (flour), fresh yeast, ground almonds	Baking powder, cake decorations, marzipan, ready to use icings, dried yeast	Batter mixes, breadcrumbs, stuffing mix

Source: Coeliacuk updated 2/15

Sources for Online Shopping

https://a2milk.co.uk
A2 milk

https://www.coeliac.org.uk/gluten-free-diet-and-lifestyle/food-and-drink-directory/
Food and drink directory suitable for Coeliacs

https://www.glutenfree-foods.co.uk/
Gluten-free foods

https://www.goodnessdirect.co.uk/
Caffeine-free, dairy-free, egg-free, gluten-free, gluten and casein-free, lactose-free, soy-free, wheat- free, yeast-free

https://www.healthyfoods-online.com/
Gluten-free, free-from

http://www.marksandspencer.com/l/food-to-order/health/gluten-free
Gluten-free available to order and collect

http://www.marksandspencer.com/l/food-to-order/health/dairy-free
Dairy-free food available to order and collect

https://www.naturalgrocery.co.uk/
Wheat-free, gluten-free, dairy-free, sugar-free

http://www.naturallygoodfood.co.uk
Gluten-free

https://www.realfoods.co.uk/
Gluten-Free, Vegan, Wheat-Free, Special Diet Food

https://www.theglutenfreekitchen.co.uk/
Free from Wheat, Dairy, Egg, Gluten, and Soya

https://www.voakesfreefrom.co.uk/

Pies, pastries, and quiches – Dairy-free, gluten-free, egg-free, soy-free

Sources for Online Information

http://cowsmilkproteinallergysupport.webs.com/free-from-foods

An up-to-date list of "free from" foods, including foods that you can find in the "normal" sections of shops and supermarkets.

https://www.glutenfreeandmore.com/

Provide a range of articles and recipe about various allergies – gluten, casein, soy, seafood, sugar, egg

Food intolerance Lab Testing (IgG)

You can arrange these through your practitioner, but if you want to go it alone both of the following UK labs have a range of tests available direct to the public:

http://www.yorktest.com
York Test

http://www.camnutri.com/
Cambridge Nutritional Sciences

Free E-Course

I know it can be hard to put information into practice sometimes, even with a book as a guide, so I've written a free e-course loaded with helpful recipes to give you a 21-day head start. Just type the following link into your browser:

https://www.oakmeadclinic.co.uk/digestive-rescue-in-just-21-days/

What Happens During a Kinesiology Consultation

During the first session, your Kinesiologist will take a full medical and lifestyle history and work with you, with your consent, to identify and address your specific individual concerns and areas causing stress.

Assessments are made using gentle manual muscle response testing where the Kinesiologist seeks to identify imbalances that may be contributing to the client's loss of health and well-being and ways to restore balance. Clients are fully clothed.

The Kinesiologist will ask you to place your arms, legs or head into specific positions and then apply light pressure against the muscle that's being tested.

Based on biofeedback from the muscle test, you and the Kinesiologist can identify precisely what is involved and devise a plan. Suggestions and advice may include incorporation of foods, nutritional supplements, relaxation and other techniques, lifestyle changes and more.

Many different factors affect and contribute to our health and well-being and using Kinesiology (manual muscle response testing) clients can be supported to come into better balance and achieve their optimum health and well-being.

Contact Details for the Association of Systematic Kinesiology:

http://www.systematic-kinesiology.co.uk/

The Principles of Functional Medicine (From the Institute for Functional Medicine)

Functional Medicine determines how and why illness occurs and restores health by addressing the root causes of disease for everyone

The Functional Medicine model is an **individualised, patient-centred, science-based approach** that empowers patients and practitioners to work together to address the underlying causes of disease and promote optimal wellness. It requires a detailed understanding of each patient's genetic, biochemical, and lifestyle factors, and leverages that data to direct personalised treatment plans that lead to improved patient outcomes.

By addressing the root cause, rather than symptoms, practitioners become oriented to identifying the complexity of disease. They may find one condition has many different causes and, likewise, one cause may result in many different conditions. As a result, Functional Medicine treatment targets the specific manifestations of disease in each individual.

All clinicians take patient history, but what makes the Functional Medicine Timeline different is that it has the effect of **giving the patient insight into previous life events** to motivate them to change and participate in treatment. As an intake tool for organising the patient's history chronologically, the Functional Medicine Timeline is a graphical representation that allows clinicians to identify factors that predispose, provoke, and contribute to pathological changes and dysfunctional responses in the patient. In this way, practitioners will be able to view temporal relationships among events, which can reveal cause-effect relationships that might otherwise go unnoticed. By covering the period from preconception to the present, the Timeline reflects the connection between the whole lifespan and one's current health.

When you visit a Functional Medicine practitioner, you can expect to spend a lot more time with them than you would with a conventional provider. You can also expect to do a lot of talking, as a large part of Functional Medicine is exploring your detailed personal and family history, the circumstances around your first symptoms, and the experiences you may have had with other healthcare providers. The

Institute for Functional Medicine teaches practitioners how to uncover the underlying causes of your health problems through careful history taking, physical examination, and laboratory testing.

By investing this time and effort up front, many people find that working with an IFM-trained provider helps them find the underlying cause of perplexing problems that have eluded other clinicians for years.

Contact details for the Institute for Functional Medicine:
https://www.ifm.org/

The Principles of Naturopathy

The Hippocratic School of Medicine first used the principles of Naturopathy in about 400 BC. The Greek philosopher Hippocrates believed in viewing the whole person in regards to finding a cause of disease and using the laws of nature to induce a cure. It was from this original school of thought that Naturopathy takes its principles [358].

- The healing power of nature - nature has the innate ability to heal

- Identify and treat the cause - there is always an underlying cause, be it physical or emotional, and this can be found by looking beyond the symptoms

- First, do no harm - a Naturopath will use the most natural, least invasive, and least toxic therapies and never use treatments that may create other conditions

- Treat the whole person - view the body as an integrated whole in all its physical and spiritual dimensions

- The Naturopath as a teacher - a Naturopath empowers the patient to take responsibility for his/her health by teaching the steps to achieve and maintain health through self-care

- Prevention is better than cure - Focus on overall health and wellness to prevent disease.

Contact details for the College of Naturopathic Medicine:

https://www.naturopathy-uk.com/

References

[1]   NHS Digital, "Health survey for England - 2013," 10 December 2014.
        [Online]. Available: http://digital.nhs.uk/catalogue/PUB16076.
        [Accessed 19 November 2017].

[2]   Allergy UK, "About Allergy," 2017. [Online]. Available:
        https://www.allergyuk.org/information-and-advice/conditions-and-
        symptoms/47-about-allergy. [Accessed 5 December 2017].

[3]   B. Nwaru, "Prevalence of common food allergies in Europe: a
        systematic review and meta-analysis," *European Journal of Allergy and
        Clinical Immunology,* vol. 69, no. 8, pp. 992-1007, 2014.

[4]   American College of Allergy, Asthma, and Autoimmunity, "Wheat
        Allergy," 2014. [Online]. Available:
        http://acaai.org/allergies/types/food-allergies/types-food-
        allergy/wheat-gluten-allergy. [Accessed 17 December 2017].

[5]   The Institute For Functional Medicine, "Adverse Food Reactions,"
        2017. [Online]. Available:
        https://functionalmedicine.widencollective.com/portals/py85vmmv/T
        oolkitAllResources. [Accessed 14 November 2017].

[6]   Allergy UK, "Why is Allergy Increasing?," September 2015. [Online].
        Available: https://www.allergyuk.org/information-and-
        advice/conditions-and-symptoms/47-about-allergy. [Accessed 4
        December 2017].

[7]   R. Gupta, "Time trends in allergic disorders in the UK," *thorax,* vol. 62,
        no. 1, pp. 91-96, 2007.

[8]   S. Benede, "The rise of food allergy: Environmental factors and
        emerging treatments," *EBioMedicine,* vol. 7, pp. 27-34, 2016.

[9]   J. Tan, "Dietary Fiber and Bacterial SCFA Enhance Oral Tolerance and
        Protect against Food Allergy through Diverse Cellular Pathways," *Cell
        Reports,* vol. 15, no. 12, pp. 2809-2824, 2016.

[10] J. Lloyd-Price, "The healthy human microbiome," *Genome Medicine,* no. 8, p. 51, 2016.

[11] C. Aranow, "Vitamin D and the Immune System," *Journal of Investigative Medicine,* vol. 59, no. 6, pp. 881-886, 2012.

[12] NHS UK, "Rickets and osteomalacia prevention," 21 December 2015. [Online]. Available: https://www.nhs.uk/conditions/rickets-and-osteomalacia/prevention/. [Accessed 4 December 2017].

[13] M. Holick, "Resurrection of vitamin D deficiency and rickets," *The Journal of Clinical Investigation,* vol. 116, no. 8, pp. 2062-2072, 2006.

[14] O. Pabst, "Oral tolerance to food protein," *Mucosal Immunology,* vol. 5, pp. 232-239, 2012.

[15] T. Paustion, "Through the Microscope 5th edn," 2009. [Online]. Available: http://www.microbiologytext.com/5th_ed/book/displayarticle/aid/393. [Accessed 14 November 2017].

[16] NHS choices, "Food Allergy," 16 May 2016. [Online]. Available: https://www.nhs.uk/conditions/food-allergy/. [Accessed 22 November 2017].

[17] Net Doctor, "EpiPen (Adrenaline)," 17 2014 June. [Online]. Available: http://www.netdoctor.co.uk/medicines/allergy-and-asthma/a6668/EpiPen-adrenaline/. [Accessed 14 November 2017].

[18] D. H. Sharma, "How Does Epinephrine turn off an allergic reaction?" 10 April 2013. [Online]. Available: https://www.allergicliving.com/experts/how-does-epinephrine-turn-off-an-allergic-reaction/. [Accessed 14 November 2017].

[19] C. Povesi, "Exercise-induced anaphylaxis: a clinical view," *Italian Journal of Paediatrics,* vol. 38, no. 43, pp. 1824-7288, 2012.

[20] B. Minty, "Food-dependent exercise-induced anaphylaxis," *The Official Journal of the College of Family Physicians of Canada,* vol. 63, no. 1, pp. 42-43, 2017.

[21]   American Academy of Allergy, Asthma and Immunology, "Allergen,"
        2017. [Online]. Available: https://www.aaaai.org/conditions-and-
        treatments/conditions-dictionary/allergen. [Accessed 21 December
        2017].

[22]   Food.Gov.UK, "Food Allergen Labelling Technical Guidance," April
        2015. [Online]. Available:
        https://www.food.gov.uk/sites/default/files/food-allergen-labelling-
        technical-guidance.pdf. [Accessed 22 December 2017].

[23]   Food.Gov.UK, "Advice on Food Allergen Labelling," November 2013.
        [Online]. Available:
        https://www.food.gov.uk/sites/default/files/multimedia/pdfs/publica
        tion/allergy-leaflet.pdf. [Accessed 14 November 2017].

[24]   H. Brough, "Dietary management of peanut and tree nut allergy: what
        exactly should patients avoid?," *Clinical and Experimental Allergy:
        Journal of the British Society for Allergy and Clinical Immunology,* vol.
        45, no. 5, pp. 859-871, 2015.

[25]   Mornflake, "Gluten Free," [Online]. Available:
        http://www.mornflake.com/our-oats/gluten-free/. [Accessed 16
        December 2017].

[26]   P. Engen, "The Gastrointestinal Microbiome: Alcohol Effects on the
        Composition of Intestinal Microbiota.," *Alcohol Research: Current
        Reviews,* vol. 37, no. 2, pp. 223-236, 2015.

[27]   E. Mutlu, "Colonic microbiome is altered in alcoholism," *American
        Journal of Physiology, Gastrointestinal and Liver Physiology,* vol. 302,
        no. 9, pp. 302-309, 2012.

[28]   W. Purves, "Why don't our digestive acids corrode our stomach
        linings?," *Scientific American,* 13 November 2001.

[29]   R. Mittal, "Transient Lower Esophageal Sphincter Relaxation,"
        Gastroenterology, vol. 109, pp. 601-610, 1995.

[30]   Harvard Medical School, "Diseases and Conditions - Gastroesophageal
        Reflux Disease Gerd," October 2014. [Online]. Available:
        https://www.health.harvard.edu/diseases-and-

conditions/gastroesophageal-reflux-disease-gerd. [Accessed 8 December 2017].

[31]   Asthma and Allergy Foundation of America, "Asthma and Gastroesophageal Reflux Disease," 2017. [Online]. Available: http://asthmaandallergies.org/asthma-allergies/asthma-and-gastroesophageal-reflux-disease/. [Accessed 8 December 2017].

[32]   H. Colledge, "Helicobacter-Pylori," 17 October 2017. [Online]. Available: https://www.healthline.com/health/helicobacter-pylori. [Accessed 5 December 2017].

[33]   C. Davis, "Helicobacter Pylori," 28 June 2016. [Online]. Available: https://www.medicinenet.com/helicobacter_pylori/article.htm. [Accessed 9 December 2017].

[34]   WebMD, "Hiatal Hernia," 2017. [Online]. Available: https://www.webmd.com/digestive-disorders/hiatal-hernia#1. [Accessed 9 December 2017].

[35]   P. Kahrilas, "Increased frequency of transient lower esophageal sphincter relaxation induced by gastric distention in reflux patients with hiatal hernia.," *Gastroenterology,* vol. 118, no. 4, pp. 688-695, 2000.

[36]   G. Karamanolis, "A glass of water immediately increases gastric pH in healthy subjects.," *Digestive Diseases and Sciences,* vol. 53, no. 12, pp. 3128-3132, 2008.

[37]   M. Feldman, "Effects of ageing and gastritis on gastric acid and pepsin secretion in humans: a prospective study.," *Gastroenterology,* vol. 110, no. 4, pp. 1043-1052, 1996.

[38]   Y. Yang, "Long-term proton pump inhibitor therapy and risk of hip fracture.," *Journal of American Medical Association,* vol. 296, no. 24, pp. 2947-2953, 2006.

[39]   D. Cerda Gabaroi, "Search for hidden secondary causes in postmenopausal women with osteoporosis," *Menopause,* vol. 17, no. 1, pp. 135-139, 2010.

[40]   Federal Drug Agency, "FDA Drug Safety Communication: Possible
        increased risk of fractures of the hip, wrist, and spine with the use of
        proton pump inhibitors," 23 May 2011. [Online]. Available:
        https://www.fda.gov/Drugs/DrugSafety/PostmarketDrugSafetyInform
        ationforPatientsandProviders/ucm213206.htm. [Accessed 9 December
        2017].

[41]   medicines and healthcare products regulatory agency, "Proton pump
        inhibitors in long-term use: reports of hypomagnesaemia," April 2012.
        [Online]. Available: https://www.gov.uk/drug-safety-update/proton-
        pump-inhibitors-in-long-term-use-reports-of-hypomagnesaemia.
        [Accessed 9 December 2017].

[42]   T. Fulop, "https://emedicine.medscape.com/article/2038394-
        treatment," 16 June 2017. [Online]. Available:
        https://emedicine.medscape.com/article/2038394-treatment.
        [Accessed 22 December 2017].

[43]   W. Gomm, "Association of Proton Pump Inhibitors With Risk of
        Dementia: A Pharmacoepidemiological Claims Data Analysis.," *Journal
        of the American Medical Association,* vol. 73, no. 4, pp. 410-416, 2016.

[44]   D. Moledina, "Proton Pump Inhibitors and CKD," *Journal of the
        American Society of Nephrology,* vol. 27, no. 10, pp. 2926-2928, 2016.

[45]   M. Boyce, "Response: a Randomised trial of the effect of a
        gastrin/CCK2 receptor antagonist on Esomeprazole-induced
        hypergastrinaemia: evidence against rebound hyperacidity," *European
        Journal of Clinical Pharmacology,* vol. 73, no. 7, p. 925, 2017.

[46]   s. R, "Gastroesophageal reflux disease-related symptom recurrence in
        patients discontinuing proton pump inhibitors for Bravo® wireless
        esophageal pH monitoring study.," *Revista de Gastroenterologia de
        Mexico,* vol. 82, no. 4, pp. 277-286, 2017.

[47]   R. Shey, "Proton-pump inhibitor therapy induces acid-related
        symptoms in healthy volunteers after withdrawal of therapy.,"
        Gastroenterology, vol. 137, no. 1, pp. 80-87, 2009.

[48]   D. Peura, "A 14-day regimen of esomeprazole 20 mg/day for frequent
        heartburn: durability of effects, symptomatic rebound, and treatment

satisfaction," *Postgraduate Medicine,* vol. 128, no. 6, pp. 577-583, 2016.

[49]   L. Pasina, "Evidence-based and unlicensed indications for proton pump inhibitors and patients' preferences for discontinuation: a pilot study in a sample of Italian community pharmacies," *Journal of Clinical Pharmacy and Therapeutics,* vol. 41, no. 2, pp. 220-223, 2016.

[50]   J. Heidelbaugh, "Proton pump inhibitors and risk of vitamin and mineral deficiency: evidence and clinical implications," *Therapeutic Advances in Drug Safety,* vol. 4, no. 3, pp. 125-133, 2013.

[51]   C. Luk, "Proton pump inhibitor-associated hypomagnesemia: what do FDA data tell us?," *The Annals of Pharmacotherapy,* vol. 47, no. 6, pp. 773-80, 2013.

[52]   N. Osterwell, "Long-Term PPI Use Associated With Low Magnesium," 7 March 2011. [Online]. Available: https://www.medscape.com/viewarticle/738230. [Accessed 10 December 2017].

[53]   D. Gracie, "The Possible Risks of Proton Pump Inhibitors," *the Medical Journal of Australia,* vol. 205, no. 7, 3 October 2016.

[54]   Y. Y, "Chronic PPI Therapy and Calcium Metabolism," *Current Gastroenterology Report,* vol. 14, no. 6, pp. 473-479, 2012.

[55]   J. Lam, "Proton pump inhibitor and histamine 2 receptor antagonist use and vitamin B12 deficiency.," *Journal of the American Medical Association,* vol. 310, no. 22, pp. 2435-2442, 2013.

[56]   C. Hutchinson, "Proton pump inhibitors suppress absorption of dietary non-haem iron in hereditary haemochromatosis," *Gut,* vol. 56, no. 9, pp. 1291-1295, 2007.

[57]   H. O'Connor, "Vitamin C in the human stomach: relation to gastric pH, gastroduodenal disease, and possible sources," *Gut,* vol. 30, pp. 436-442, 1989.

[58]   C. Farrell, "Proton Pump Inhibitors Interfere With Zinc Absorption and Zinc Body Stores," *Gastroenterology Research,* vol. 4, no. 6, p. 243–251, 2011.

[59]   R. Urbas, "Malabsorption-Related Issues Associated with Chronic Proton Pump Inhibitor Usage," *Austin Journal of Nutrition and Metabolism,* vol. 3, no. 2, p. 1041, 2016.

[60]   J. Thiesen, "Suppression of gastric acid secretion in patients with gastroesophageal reflux disease results in gastric bacterial overgrowth and deconjugation of bile acids.," *Journal of Gastrointestinal Surgery,* vol. 4, no. 1, pp. 50-54, 2000.

[61]   S. Vakevainen, "Hypochlorhydria induced by a proton pump inhibitor leads to intragastric microbial production of acetaldehyde from ethanol.," *Alimentary Pharmacology & Therapeutics,* vol. 14, no. 11, pp. 1511-1518, 2000.

[62]   Pancreatic Cancer Action Network, "Pancreatic Enzymes," 2017. [Online]. Available: https://www.pancan.org/facing-pancreatic-cancer/diet-and-nutrition/pancreatic-enzymes/. [Accessed 5 December 2017].

[63]   A. Fieker, "Enzyme replacement therapy for pancreatic insufficiency: present and future," *Clinical and Experimental Gastroenterology,* vol. 4, pp. 55-73, 2011.

[64]   M. DeMeo, "Intestinal permeation and gastrointestinal disease.," *Journal of Clinical Gastroenterology,* vol. 34, no. 4, pp. 385-396, 2002.

[65]   S. Bischoff, "Intestinal permeability – a new target for disease prevention and therapy," *Gastroenterology,* vol. 14, p. 189, 2014.

[66]   A. Fasano, "Zonulin and Its Regulation of Intestinal Barrier Function: The Biological Door to Inflammation, Autoimmunity, and Cancer," *Physiological Reviews,* vol. 91, no. 1, pp. 151-175, 2011.

[67]   A. Lerner, "Changes in intestinal tight junction permeability associated with industrial food additives explain the rising incidence of

autoimmune disease," *Autoimmunity Reviews,* vol. 14, no. 6, pp. 479-489, June 2015.

[68]   D. Duerksen, "A Comparison of Antibody Testing, Permeability Testing, and Zonulin Levels with Small-Bowel Biopsy in Celiac Disease Patients on a Gluten-Free Diet," *Digestive Diseases and Sciences,* vol. 55, no. 4, p. 1026–1031 |, 2010.

[69]   T. Jalonen, "Identical intestinal permeability changes in children with different clinical manifestations of cow's milk allergy," *Journal of Allergy and Clinical Immunology,* vol. 88, no. 5, pp. 737-742, 1991.

[70]   I. Bjarnason, "Effect of non-steroidal anti-inflammatory drugs and prostaglandins on the permeability of the human small intestine.," *Gut,* vol. 27, no. 11, p. 1292–1297, 1986.

[71]   E. Smecuol, "Acute gastrointestinal permeability responses to different non-steroidal anti-inflammatory drugs," *Gut,* vol. 49, no. 5, p. 650–655, 2001.

[72]   L. Zuo, "Cigarette smoking is associated with intestinal barrier dysfunction in the small intestine but not in the large intestine of mice," *Journal of Crohn's and Colitis,* vol. 8, no. 12, p. 1710–1722, 2014.

[73]   Y. Yang, "Effects of alcohol on intestinal epithelial barrier permeability and expression of tight junction-associated proteins.," *Molecular Medicine Reports,* vol. 9, no. 6, pp. 2352-2356, 2014.

[74]   A. Lerner, "Changes in intestinal tight junction permeability associated with industrial food additives explain the rising incidence of autoimmune disease," *Autoimmunity Reviews,* vol. 14, no. 6, pp. 479-489, 2015.

[75]   Coeliac UK, "About Coeliac disease: genetics," [Online]. Available: https://www.coeliac.org.uk/coeliac-disease/about-coeliac-disease-and-dermatitis-herpetiformis/genetics/. [Accessed 28 November 2017].

[76]   V. d. Broeck, "Presence of celiac disease epitopes in modern and old hexaploid wheat varieties: wheat breeding may have contributed to

increased prevalence of celiac disease," *Theoretical and Applied Genetics,* vol. 121, no. 8, p. 1527–1539, 2010.

[77] U. Ghoshal, "Partially responsive celiac disease resulting from small intestinal bacterial overgrowth and lactose intolerance.," *BMC Gastroenterology,* vol. 4, p. 10, 2004.

[78] K. Garsed, "Can oats be taken in a gluten-free diet? A systematic review," *Scandinavian Journal of Gastroenterology,* vol. 42, no. 2, pp. 171-178, 2009.

[79] E. J. Hoffenberg, "A trial of oats in children with newly diagnosed celiac disease," *The Journal of Pediatrics,* vol. 137, no. 3, pp. 361-366, 2000.

[80] K. Lundin, "Oats induced villous atrophy in coeliac disease," *BMJ Journals,* vol. 52, no. 11, 2003.

[81] J. Ludviggson, "Diagnosis and management of adult coeliac disease: guidelines from the British Society of Gastroenterology," *Gut,* vol. 63, pp. 1210-1228, 2014.

[82] Gluten Intolerance Group, "Nutritional Deficiencies in Celiac Disease and Non-Celiac Gluten Sensitivity," 10 May 2017. [Online]. Available: https://www.gluten.org/resources/diet-nutrition/nutrient-deficiencies/. [Accessed 30 November 2017].

[83] U. Volta, "Non-celiac gluten sensitivity: questions still to be answered despite increasing awareness," *Cellular & Molecular Immunology,* vol. 10, no. 5, pp. 383-392, 2013.

[84] A. Sapone, "Differential Mucosal IL-17 Expression in Two Gliadin-Induced Disorders: Gluten Sensitivity and the Autoimmune Enteropathy Celiac Disease," *International Archives of Allergy and Immunology,* vol. 152, no. 75, pp. 75-80, 2010.

[85] U. Volta, "Serological Tests in Gluten Sensitivity (Nonceliac Gluten Intolerance)," *Journal of Clinical Gastroenterology,* vol. 46, no. 8, pp. 680-685, 2012.

[86]   United States Department of Agriculture, "World Wheat Production 2017/18," June 2017. [Online]. Available: https://www.worldwheatproduction.com/. [Accessed 23 December 2017].

[87]   Food and Agriculture Association of the United Nations, "World Food Situation," 7 December 2017. [Online]. Available: http://www.fao.org/worldfoodsituation/csdb/en/. [Accessed 23 December 2017].

[88]   H. McGee, On Food and Cooking. The Science of Lore of the Kitchen, Simon and Schuster, 1984.

[89]   S. Fallon, Nourishing Traditions, New Trends Publishing, 2000.

[90]   Rothamsted Research, "Broadwalk winter Wheat Experiment," 2017. [Online]. Available: http://www.era.rothamsted.ac.uk/index.php?area=home&page=index&dataset=4. [Accessed 17 December 2017].

[91]   P. Shewry, "The structure and properties of gluten: an elastic protein from wheat grain," *Philosophical Transactions of the Royal Society B London Biological Sciences,* vol. 357, p. 133–142, 2002.

[92]   M. Fan, "Evidence of decreasing mineral density in wheat grain over the last 160 years," *Journal of Trace Elements in Medicine and Biology,* vol. 22, no. 4, pp. 315-324, 2008.

[93]   F. Zhao, "Variation in mineral micronutrient concentrations in grain of wheat lines of diverse origin," *Journal of Cereal Science,* vol. 49, no. 2, pp. 290-295, 2009.

[94]   M. McMullen, "Seed Treatment for Disease Control," March 2000. [Online]. Available: https://library.ndsu.edu/ir/bitstream/handle/10365/9120/PP447_2000.pdf?sequence=1&isAllowed=y. [Accessed 23 December 2017].

[95]   Agriculture and Horticulture Development Management Board, "HGCA Wheat disease and Management Guide 2012," Spring 2012. [Online]. Available:

http://adlib.everysite.co.uk/resources/000/160/665/G54_Wheat_dise
ase_management_guide_2012.pdf. [Accessed 23 December 2017].

[96]   G. Seralini, "RETRACTED: Long term toxicity of a Roundup herbicide
       and a Roundup-tolerant genetically modified maize," *Food and
       Chemical Toxicology,* vol. 50, no. 11, pp. 4221-4231, 2012.

[97]   G. Seralini, "Answers to critics: Why there is long term toxicity due to a
       Roundup-tolerant genetically modified maize and to a Roundup
       herbicide," *Food and Chemical Toxicology,* vol. 53, pp. 476-483, 2013.

[98]   Wikipedia, "The Seralini Affair," [Online]. Available:
       https://en.wikipedia.org/wiki/S%C3%A9ralini_affair. [Accessed 23
       December 2017].

[99]   C. Snell, "Assessment of the health impact of GM plant diets in long-
       term and multigenerational animal feeding trials: A literature review,"
       Food and Chemical Toxicology, vol. 50, no. 3-4, pp. 1134-1148, 2012.

[100] G. Sertoli, "Roundup disrupts male reproductive functions by
       triggering calcium-mediated cell death in rat testis and Sertoli cells,"
       Free Radical Biology and Medicine, vol. 65, pp. 335-346, 2013.

[101] V. Cavalli, "Roundup disrupts male reproductive functions by
       triggering calcium-mediated cell death in rat testis and Sertoli cells,"
       Free Radical Biology and Medicine, vol. 65, pp. 335-346, 2013.

[102] E. Cassault-Meyer, "An acute exposure to glyphosate-based herbicide
       alters aromatase levels in testis and sperm nuclear quality,"
       Environmental Toxicology and Pharmacology, vol. 38, no. 1, pp. 131-
       140, 2014.

[103] E. Clair, "A glyphosate-based herbicide induces necrosis and apoptosis
       in mature rat testicular cells in vitro, and testosterone decrease at
       lower levels," *Toxicology in Vitro,* vol. 26, no. 2, pp. 269-279, 2012.

[104] C. Heu, "A step further toward glyphosate-induced epidermal cell
       death: Involvement of mitochondrial and oxidative mechanisms,"
       Environmental Toxicology and Pharmacology, vol. 34, no. 2, pp. 144-
       153, 2012.

[105] M. Chlopecka, "Glyphosate affects the spontaneous motoric activity of intestine at very low doses – In vitro study," *Pesticide Biochemistry and Physiology,* vol. 113, pp. 25-30, 2014.

[106] C. Gasnier, "Glyphosate-based herbicides are toxic and endocrine disruptors in human cell lines.," *Toxicology,* vol. 262, no. 3, pp. 184-91, 2009.

[107] D. Cressey, "https://www.scientificamerican.com/article/widely-used-herbicide-linked-to-cancer/," *Scientific American,* 25 March 2015.

[108] C. Hogue, "California to list glyphosate as a carcinogen," *Chemical & Engineering News,* vol. 95, no. 27, p. 14, July 2017.

[109] D. Pizzuti, "Lack of intestinal mucosal toxicity of Triticum monococcum in celiac disease patients," *Scandinavian Journal of Gastroenterology,* vol. 41, no. 11, pp. 1305-1311, 2006.

[110] M. Pietzak, "Celiac Disease, Wheat Allergy, and Gluten Sensitivity," *Journal of Parenteral and Enteral Nutrition,* vol. 36, no. 1, p. Supplemental, 2012.

[111] M. Vazquez-Roque, "A Controlled Trial of Gluten-Free Diet in Patients With Irritable Bowel Syndrome-Diarrhea: Effects on Bowel Frequency and Intestinal Function," *Gastroenterology,* vol. 144, no. 5, pp. 903-911, 2013.

[112] K. Parameswaran, "Changes in the carbohydrates and nitrogenous components during germination of proso millet, Panicum miliaceum," *Plant Foods for Human Nutrition,* vol. 45, no. 2, pp. 97-102, 1994.

[113] F. Yang, "Studies on germination conditions and antioxidant contents of wheat grain," *International Journal of Food Sciences and Nutrition,* vol. 52, no. 4, pp. 319-330, 2001.

[114] P. Koehler, "Changes of folates, dietary fibre, and proteins in wheat as affected by germination," *Journal of Agricultural and Food Chemistry,* vol. 55, no. 12, pp. 4678-4683, 2007.

[115] A. Akobeng, "Systematic review: tolerable amount of gluten for people with coeliac disease.," *Alimentary Pharmacology & Therapeutics,* vol. 27, no. 11, pp. 1044-1052, 2008.

[116] Coeliac UK, "The Gluten-Free Diet - Grains," [Online]. Available: https://www.coeliac.org.uk/gluten-free-diet-and-lifestyle/gf-diet/grains/. [Accessed 22 November 2017].

[117] M. Pastore, "Six Months of Gluten-Free Diet Don't Influence Autoantibody Titers, but Improve Insulin Secretion in Subjects at High Risk for Type 1 Diabetes," *The Journal of Clinical Endocrinology & Metabolism,* vol. 88, no. 1, p. 162–165, 2003.

[118] G. De Palma, "Effects of a gluten-free diet on gut microbiota and immune function in healthy adult human subjects.," *British Journal of Nutrition,* vol. 102, no. 8, pp. 1154-1160, 2010.

[119] F. He, "Increased consumption of fruit and vegetables is related to a reduced risk of coronary heart disease: a meta-analysis of cohort studies," *Journal of Human Hypertension,* vol. 21, p. 717–728, 2007.

[120] R. Hai Liu, "Health-Promoting Components of Fruits and Vegetables in the Diet," *Advances in Nutrition,* vol. 4, pp. 384S-392S, 2013.

[121] G. Ruel, "Association between nutrition and the evolution of multimorbidity: The importance of fruits and vegetables and whole grain products," *Clinical Nutrition,* vol. 33, no. 3, pp. 513-520, 2014.

[122] A. Abdel-Haleem, "Producing of Gluten- Free and Casein Free (GFCF) Cupcakes for Autistic Children," *Journal of Food and Nutrition Disorders,* vol. 4, no. 3, 2015.

[123] K. Reichelt, "Probable aetiology and possible treatment of childhood autism," *American Psychological Association,* vol. 4, no. 6, pp. 308-319, 1991.

[124] A. Knivsberg, "A randomised, controlled study of dietary intervention in autistic syndromes.," *Nutrritional Neuroscience,* vol. 5, no. 4, pp. 251-61, 2002.

[125] N. Salvatori, " Asthma induced by inhalation of flour in adults with food allergy to wheat," *Clinical and Experimental Allergy,* vol. 38, no. 8, pp. 1349-1356, 2008.

[126] H. Ramesh, "Food allergy overview in children," *Clinical Reviews in Allergy & Immunology,* vol. 34, no. 2, pp. 217-230, 2008.

[127] H. Matsuo, "Sensitivity and specificity of recombinant omega-5 gliadin-specific IgE measurement for the diagnosis of wheat-dependent exercise-induced anaphylaxis," *Allergy,* vol. 63, no. 2, pp. 233-236, 2008.

[128] U.S. National Library of Medicine, "What is a gene?," 19 December 2017. [Online]. Available: https://ghr.nlm.nih.gov/primer/basics/gene. [Accessed 23 December 2017].

[129] U.S. National Library of Medicine Genetics Home Reference, "FLG gene," 19 December 2017. [Online]. Available: https://ghr.nlm.nih.gov/gene/FLG. [Accessed 23 December 2017].

[130] U.S. National Library of Medicine, "FLG gene," December 2017. [Online]. Available: https://ghr.nlm.nih.gov/gene/FLG. [Accessed 13 December 2017].

[131] A. Linneburg, "Association between Loss-of-Function Mutations in the Filaggrin Gene and Self-Reported Food Allergy and Alcohol Sensitivity," *International Archives of Allergy and Immunology,* vol. 161, pp. 234-242, 2013.

[132] R. Kopec, "Avocado consumption enhances human postprandial provitamin A absorption and conversion from a novel high-β-carotene tomato sauce and from carrots.," *Journal of Nutrition,* vol. 144, no. 8, pp. 1158-1166, 2014.

[133] N. Unlu, "Carotenoid absorption from salad and salsa by humans is enhanced by the addition of avocado or avocado oil.," *Journal of Nutrition,* vol. 135, no. 3, pp. 431-6, 2005.

[134] V. Fulgoni, "Avocado consumption is associated with better diet quality and nutrient intake, and lower metabolic syndrome risk in US adults: results from the National Health and Nutrition Examination

Survey (NHANES) 2001-2008," *Nutrition Journal,* vol. 12, no. 1, pp. 1475-2891, 2013.

[135] Z. Pieterze, "Substitution of high monounsaturated fatty acid avocado for mixed dietary fats during an energy-restricted diet: effects on weight loss, serum lipids, fibrinogen, and vascular function.," *Nutrition,* vol. 21, no. 1, pp. 67-75, 2005.

[136] G. Donnarumma, "AV119, a natural sugar from avocado gratissima, modulates the LPS-induced proinflammatory response in human keratinocytes.," *Inflammation,* vol. 34, no. 6, pp. 568-575, 2011.

[137] G. Mateljan, "the World's Healthiest Foods - Avocados," 2017. [Online]. Available: http://whfoods.org/genpage.php?tname=foodspice&dbid=5. [Accessed 6 December 2017].

[138] E. Carey, "How to Cope With An Avocado Allergy," 17 March 2015. [Online]. Available: https://www.healthline.com/health/food-nutrition/how-to-cope-with-an-avocado-allergy#3. [Accessed 23 December 2017].

[139] Mintel, "Brits carve their meat intake: 28% of Brits have cut back their meat consumption over the last six months," 9 August 2017. [Online]. Available: http://www.mintel.com/press-centre/food-and-drink/28-of-brits-have-cut-back-their-meat-consumption-over-the-last-six-months. [Accessed 5 December 2017].

[140] G. Mateljan, "World's Healthiest Foods - Beef, grass-fed," 2017. [Online]. Available: http://whfoods.org/genpage.php?tname=foodspice&dbid=141. [Accessed 5 December 2017].

[141] S. Van Nunen, "An association between tick bite reactions and red meat allergy in humans.," *The Medical Journal of Australia,* vol. 190, no. 9, pp. 510-511, 2009.

[142] J. Steinke, "The alpha-gal story: Lessons learned from connecting the dots," *The Journal of Allergy and Clinical Immunology,* vol. 135, no. 3, pp. 589-597, 2015.

[143] S. Commins, "Delayed Anaphylaxis to Red Meat in Patients with IgE Specific for Galactose alpha-1,3-Galactose (alpha-gal)," *Current Allergy and Asthma Reports,* vol. 13, no. 1, pp. 72-77, 2013.

[144] B. Ballmer-Weber, "Celery allergy confirmed by double-blind, placebo-controlled food challenge: a clinical study in 32 subjects with a history of adverse reactions to celery root.," *Journal of Allergy and Clinical Immunology,* vol. 106, no. 2, pp. 373-378, 2000.

[145] M. Ashwood-smith, "Mechanism of photosensitivity reactions to diseased celery.," *British Medical Journal,* p. 1249, 27 April 1985.

[146] S. Chaudhary, "Increased furocoumarin content of celery during storage," *Journal of Agricultural and Food Chemistry,* vol. 33, no. 6, pp. 1153-1157, November 1985.

[147] Anaphylaxis.org.uk, "Celery Allergy: the Facts," December 2014. [Online]. Available: ttps://www.anaphylaxis.org.uk/wp-content/uploads/2015/06/Celery-version-9-formatted-with-changes-to-terminology-re-pollen-food.pdf. [Accessed 14 November 2017].

[148] NHS choices, "Scurvy," 15 September 2017. [Online]. Available: https://www.nhs.uk/conditions/scurvy/. [Accessed 11 December 2017].

[149] N. Naganuma, "A study of the phototoxicity of lemon oil.," *Archives of Dermatological Research,* vol. 278, no. 1, pp. 31-36, 1985.

[150] J. Thomson, "There's A Huge Difference Between The Corn We Eat vs What Cows Eat," 20 July 2017. [Online]. Available: http://www.huffingtonpost.co.uk/entry/sweet-corn-vs-field-corn_us_596f6718e4b0a03aba868f75. [Accessed 11 December 2017].

[151] G. Mateljan, "Corn, Fresh Sweet," 2017. [Online]. Available: http://whfoods.org/genpage.php?tname=foodspice&dbid=90. [Accessed 11 December 2017].

[152] WebMD, "Corn silk," 2009. [Online]. Available: https://www.webmd.com/vitamins-supplements/ingredientmono-140-

corn%20silk.aspx?activeingredientid=140&activeingredientname=corn
%20silk. [Accessed 11 December 2017].

[153] Toxinology.no, "Crustacean Allergies," 2010. [Online]. Available:
http://toxinology.nilu.no/Researchareas/Foodallergens/Factsheets/Cr
ustaceanallergy.aspx. [Accessed 3 December 2017].

[154] K. James, "Shellfish toxicity: human health implications of marine algal
toxins," *Epidemiol. Infect.,* vol. 138, no. 7, pp. 927-940, 2010.

[155] C. Woo, "Not all shellfish "allergy" is allergy!," *Clinical and
Translational Allergy,* vol. 1, no. 3, pp. 2045-7022, June.

[156] Egg nutrition Center.Org, "Eggs - Fascinating Facts," [Online].
Available: http://thinkegg.com/index.php/21-2/. [Accessed 10
december 2017].

[157] M. Fernandez, "Rethinking dietary cholesterol.," *Current Opinion in
Clinical Nutrition and Metabolic Care,* vol. 15, no. 2, pp. 117-21, 2012.

[158] K. Herron, "High intake of cholesterol results in less atherogenic low-
density lipoprotein particles in men and women independent of
response classification," *Journal of the American Medical Association,*
vol. 53, no. 6, pp. 823-830, 2004.

[159] P. Jones, "Dietary Cholesterol Feeding Suppresses Human Cholesterol
Synthesis Measured by Deuterium Incorporation and Urinary
Mevalonic Acid Levels," *Arteriosclerosis, Thrombosis and Vascular
Biology,* vol. 16, pp. 1222-1228, 1996.

[160] C. Packard, "The role of small, dense low-density lipoprotein (LDL): a
new look," *International Journal of Cardiology,* vol. 74, no. 1, pp. S17-
S22, 2000.

[161] P. Schnoor, "Egg consumption and high-density-lipoprotein
cholesterol.," *Journal of Internal Medicine,* vol. 235, no. 3, pp. 249-51,
1994.

[162] S. Kritchevsky, "A Review of Scientific Research and Recommendations
Regarding Eggs," *Journal of the American College of Nutrition,* vol. 23,
no. S6, pp. 596S-600S, 2004.

[163] M. Flynn, "Effect of dietary egg on human serum cholesterol and triglycerides.," *American Journal of Clinical Nutrition,* vol. 32, no. 5, pp. 1051-1057, 1979.

[164] The University of Wisconsin Health, "Health Facts for You - Egg Allergy Diet," October 2015. [Online]. Available: https://www.uwhealth.org/healthfacts/nutrition/270.pdf. [Accessed 30 November 2017].

[165] The Mayo Clinic, "Diseases and Conditions: Egg Allergy," 27 Jan 2015. [Online]. Available: https://www.mayoclinic.org/diseases-conditions/egg-allergy/basics/prevention/con-20032721. [Accessed 30 November 2017].

[166] American College of Allergy, Asthma, & Immunology, "Egg Allergy," 2014. [Online]. Available: http://acaai.org/allergies/types/food-allergies/types-food-allergy/egg-allergy. [Accessed 29 November 2017].

[167] Food and Agriculture Organization of the United Nations, "Nature's Superfood: 10 Interesting Facts on Fish and Nutrition," 30 2015 September. [Online]. Available: http://www.fao.org/home/en/. [Accessed 7 December 2017].

[168] American College of Allergy, Asthma and Immunology, "Fish Allergy," 2014. [Online]. Available: http://acaai.org/allergies/types/food-allergies/types-food-allergy/fish-allergy. [Accessed 2 December 2017].

[169] European Centre for Allergy Research Foundation, "Fish Allergy," July 2016. [Online]. Available: http://www.ecarf.org/en/information-portal/allergies-overview/fish-allergy/. [Accessed 2 December 2017].

[170] Food Allergy Research & Education, "Food Allergens in Medications," 16 June 2014. [Online]. Available: https://www.foodallergy.org/about-fare/blog/food-allergens-in-medications. [Accessed 2 December 2017].

[171] E. Vassilopoulou, "Risk of allergic reactions to wine, in milk, egg and fish-allergic patients," *Clinical and Translational Allergy,* vol. 1, no. 10, 2011.

[172] D. Ong, "Manipulation of dietary short chain carbohydrates alters the pattern of gas production and genesis of symptoms in irritable bowel syndrome.," *Journal of Gastroenterology and Hepatology,* vol. 25, no. 8, pp. 1366-1373, 2010.

[173] L. Marciani, "Postprandial Changes in Small Bowel Water Content in Healthy Subjects and Patients With Irritable Bowel Syndrome," *Gastroenterology,* vol. 138, no. 2, p. 469–477.e1, 2010.

[174] H. Staudacher, "Comparison of symptom response following advice for a diet low in fermentable carbohydrates (FODMAPs) versus standard dietary advice in patients with irritable bowel syndrome," *Journal of Human Nutrition and Dietetics,* vol. 24, no. 5, p. 487–495, 2011.

[175] P. Gibson, "Food Choice as a Key Management Strategy for Functional Gastrointestinal Symptoms," *The American Journal of Gastroenterology,* vol. 107, p. 657–666, 2012.

[176] P. Gibson, "Evidence-based dietary management of functional gastrointestinal symptoms: The FODMAP approach," *Journal of Gastroenterology and Hepatology,* vol. 25, no. 2, p. 252–258, 2009.

[177] S. Shepherd, "Short-Chain Carbohydrates and Functional Gastrointestinal Disorders," *American Journal of Gastroenterology,* vol. 108, p. 707–717, 2013.

[178] S. Shepherd, "Fructose Malabsorption and Symptoms of Irritable Bowel Syndrome: Guidelines for Effective Dietary Management," *Journal of the American Dietetic Association,* vol. 106, no. 10, pp. 1631-1639, 2006.

[179] J. Valdez-Palomares, "Low FODMAPs Diet Increases the Abundance of Bifidobacterium in Mexican Patients with Irritable Bowel Syndrome," *The Official Journal of the Federation of American Societies for Experimental Biology,* vol. 31, no. 1, p. 968.9, 2017.

[180] K. Muhammad Nawawi, "PTU-124 Low fodmaps diet significantly improves IBS symptoms: an Irish retrospective cohort study," *British Medical Journal, Gut,* vol. 66, no. 2, 2017.

[181] M. Zahedi, "Low FODMAPs diet vs general dietary advice improves clinical response in patients with diarrhea-predominant irritable bowel syndrome: a randomized controlled trial," *The Journal of Gastroenterology and Hepatology,* 2017.

[182] the Food and Drug Administration, "Fish and Fishery Products Hazards and Controls Guidance - Fourth Edition," 11 November 2017. [Online]. Available: https://www.fda.gov/downloads/Food/GuidanceRegulation/UCM252 400.pdf. [Accessed 23 December 2017].

[183] Atuna.com, "Histamine (Scombrotoxin)," 2017. [Online]. Available: http://www.atuna.com/index.php/en/health/histamine. [Accessed 23 December 2017].

[184] D. Freed, "Do dietary lectins cause disease? The evidence is suggestive—and raises interesting possibilities for treatment ," *BMJ,* vol. 318, pp. 1023-1024, 1999.

[185] E. Lipski, "Food Sensitivities, Intolerances, Allergies. 4 Edn," in *Digestive Wellness*, New York, McGraw-Hill, 2012, p. 157.

[186] L. Cordain, "Modulation of immune function by dietary lectins in rheumatoid arthritis," *British Journal of Nutrition,* vol. 83, no. 3, pp. 207-217, 2007.

[187] A. Vojdani, "Lectins, agglutinins, and their roles in autoimmune reactivities," *Alternative Therapies in Health and Medicine,* vol. 21, no. Supplement 1, pp. 46-51, 2015.

[188] J. Rodhouse, "Red kidney bean poisoning in the UK: an analysis of 50 suspected incidents between 1976 and 1989.," *Epidemiology and Infection,* vol. 105, no. 3, pp. 485-491, 1990.

[189] A. Iqbal, "Nutritional quality of important food legumes," *Food Chemistry,* vol. 97, no. 2, pp. 331-335, 2006.

[190] M. Messina, "Legumes and soybeans: an overview of their nutritional profiles and health effects," *American Society for Clinical Nutrition,* vol. 70, no. 3, pp. 439-450, 1999.

[191] USA Emergency Supplies, "All About Beans And Legumes," 2017. [Online]. Available: //www.usaemergencysupply.com/information-center/all-about/all-about-beans-and-legumes. [Accessed 5 December 2017].

[192] J. Crespo, "Frequency of food allergy in a pediatric population from Spain," *Paediatric Allergy and Immunology,* vol. 6, no. 1, pp. 39-43, 1995.

[193] Wikipedia, "Lupinus," 16 December 2017. [Online]. Available: https://en.wikipedia.org/wiki/Lupinus. [Accessed 23 December 2017].

[194] M. Mennini, "Lupin and Other Potentially Cross-Reactive Allergens in Peanut Allergy.," *Current Allergy & Asthma Reports,* vol. 16, no. 12, p. November 2016.

[195] A. S. B. e. at, "Variably severe systemic allergic reactions after consuming foods with unlabelled lupin flour: a case series," 16 February 2014. [Online]. Available: https://jmedicalcasereports.biomedcentral.com/articles/10.1186/175 2-1947-8-55. [Accessed 14 November 2017].

[196] J. Burger, "Absence of the lactase-persistence-associated allele in early Neolithic Europeans," *Journal of the National Academy of Sciences of the United States,* vol. 104, no. 10, p. 3736–3741, 27 December 2006.

[197] A. Bate, "UK Dairy Industry Statistics, House of Common Briefing Paper No 2721," 20 January 2016. [Online]. Available: researchbriefings.files.parliament.uk/documents/SN02721/SN02721.p df. [Accessed 16 December 2017].

[198] Compassion in World Farming, "About Dairy Cows," 2017. [Online]. Available: https://www.ciwf.org.uk/farm-animals/cows/dairy-cows/. [Accessed 16 December 2017].

[199] U.S. Food and Drug Administration, "Bovine Somatotropin (BST)," 27 October 2017. [Online]. Available: https://www.fda.gov/AnimalVeterinary/SafetyHealth/ProductSafetyIn formation/ucm055435.htm. [Accessed 23 December 2017].

[200] D. Brinckman, "The Regulation Of rBST: The European Case," *The Journal of Agrobiotechnology Management And Economics,* vol. 3, no. 2 and 3, p. Article 15, 2000.

[201] P. Sebeley, "Milk Intolerance, Beta-Casein and Lactose," *Nutrients,* vol. 7, no. 9, p. 7285–7297, 2015.

[202] G. Mateljan, "Calcium," 2017. [Online]. Available: http://whfoods.org/genpage.php?tname=nutrient&dbid=45. [Accessed 16 December 2017].

[203] "Lifetime high calcium intake increases osteoporotic fracture risk in old age," *Medical Hypotheses,* vol. 65, no. 3, pp. 552-558, 2005.

[204] A. Lanou, "Should dairy be recommended as part of a healthy vegetarian diet? Counterpoint.," *The American Journal of Clinical Nutrition,* vol. 89, no. 5, pp. 1638S-1642S, 2009.

[205] Y. Song, "Whole milk intake is associated with prostate cancer-specific mortality among U.S. male physicians," *The Journal of Nutrition,* vol. 143, no. 2, pp. 189-96, 2013.

[206] Q. LQ, "Milk consumption and circulating insulin-like growth factor-I level: a systematic literature review," *International Journal of Food Sciences and Nutrition,* vol. 60, no. Suppl 7, pp. 330-340, 2009.

[207] D. Felson, "Effects of weight and body mass index on bone mineral density in men and women: The Framingham study," *The American Society for Bone and Mineral Research,* vol. 8, no. 5, p. 567–573, 1993.

[208] R. Rizzoli, "The role of dietary protein and vitamin D in maintaining musculoskeletal health in postmenopausal women: A consensus statement from the European Society for Clinical and Economic Aspects of Osteoporosis and Osteoarthritis (ESCEO)," *Maturitas,* vol. 79, no. 1, pp. 122-132, 2014.

[209] F. Zhang, "Vitamin D Deficiency Is Associated with Progression of Knee Osteoarthritis," *The Journal of Nutrition,* vol. 144, no. 12, pp. 2002-2008, 2014.

[210] G. Iolascon, "Vitamin D supplementation in a fractured patient: how, when and why," *Clinical Cases in Mineral and Bone Metabolism,* vol. 6, no. 2, p. 120–124, 2009.

[211] T. Vesa, "Tolerance to small amounts of lactose in lactose maldigesters.," *American Journal of Clinical Nutrition,* vol. 64, no. 2, pp. 197-201, 1996.

[212] R. Canani, "Diagnosing and Treating Intolerance to Carbohydrates in Children," *Nutrients,* vol. 8, no. 3, p. 157, 2016.

[213] S. Tishkoff, "Convergent adaptation of human lactase persistence in Africa and Europe.," *Nature Genetics,* vol. 39, no. 1, pp. 31-40, 2007.

[214] The Tech Museum of Innovation, Stanford School of Medicine, "Milk and the Modern Man - the rise of adult milk drinking," 2013. [Online]. Available: http://genetics.thetech.org/original_news/news45. [Accessed 24 December 2017].

[215] D. Swallow, "Genetics of lactase persistence and lactose intolerance.," *Annual Review of Genetics,* vol. 37, pp. 197-219, 2003.

[216] B. R, "Lactose Intolerance (Lactase Non-Persistence)," [Online]. Available: http://www.vivo.colostate.edu/hbooks/pathphys/digestion/smallgut/lactose_intol.html. [Accessed 4 December 2017].

[217] M. Ul Haq, "Consumption of β-casomorphins-7/5 induce an inflammatory immune response in mice gut through the Th2 pathway," *Journal of Functional Foods,* vol. 8, pp. 150-160, 2014.

[218] M. Barnett, "Dietary A1 β-casein affects gastrointestinal transit time, dipeptidyl peptidase-4 activity, and inflammatory status relative to A2 β-casein in Wistar rats," *International Journal of Food Sciences and Nutrition,* vol. 65, no. 6, pp. 720-727, 2014.

[219] M. Ul Haq, "Comparative evaluation of cow β-casein variants (A1/A2) consumption on the Th2-mediated inflammatory response in mouse gut," *European Journal of Nutrition,* vol. 53, no. 4, pp. 1039-1049, 2014.

[220] S. Ho, "Comparative effects of A1 versus A2 beta-casein on gastrointestinal measures: a blinded randomised cross-over pilot study," *European Journal of Clinical Nutrition,* vol. 68, no. 9, pp. 994-1000, 2014.

[221] N. Kost, "Beta-casomorphins-7 in infants on different type of feeding and different levels of psychomotor development," *Peptides,* vol. 30, no. 10, pp. 1854-1860, 2009.

[222] O. Sokolov, "Autistic children display elevated urine levels of bovine casomorphin-7 immunoreactivity," *Peptides,* vol. 56, no. 68, pp. 68-71, 2014.

[223] J. Chia, "A1 beta-casein milk protein and other environmental pre-disposing factors for type 1 diabetes," *Nutrition and Diabetes,* vol. 7, no. 5, p. e274, 2017.

[224] S. Jianqin, "Effects of milk containing only A2 beta casein versus milk containing both A1 and A2 beta-casein proteins on gastrointestinal physiology, symptoms of discomfort, and cognitive behavior of people with self-reported intolerance to traditional cows' milk," *Nutrition Journal,* vol. 15, p. 45, 2016.

[225] K. Tailford, "A casein variant in cow's milk is atherogenic," *Atherosclerosis,* vol. 170, no. 1, pp. 13-9, 2003.

[226] L. Pelto, "Milk hypersensitivity--key to poorly defined gastrointestinal symptoms in adults.," *Allergy,* vol. 53, no. 3, pp. 307-310, 1998.

[227] J. Bartley, "Does milk increase mucus production?," *Medical Hypotheses,* vol. 74, no. 4, pp. 732-734, 2010.

[228] R. Crittenden, "Cow's milk allergy: a complex disorder," *Jounal of the American College of Nutrition,* vol. 24, no. 6, pp. 582S-91S, 2005.

[229] Tetra-pak, "Cheese Making," 2015. [Online]. Available: http://dairyprocessinghandbook.com/chapter/cheese. [Accessed 17 December 2017].

[230] D. Nguyen, "Formation and Degradation of Beta-casomorphins in Dairy Processing," *Critical Reviews in Food Science and Nutrition,* vol. 55, no. 14, pp. 1955-1967, 2015.

[231] Self nutrition Data, "Butter," 2014. [Online]. Available: http://nutritiondata.self.com/facts/dairy-and-egg-products/133/2. [Accessed 30 December 2017].

[232] The Dairy Council, "Yogurt Factsheet," January 2017. [Online]. Available: https://www.milk.co.uk/hcp/wp-content/uploads/sites/2/woocommerce_uploads/2016/12/Yogurt-factsheet-2017.pdf. [Accessed 30 December 2017].

[233] O. Adolfsson, "Yogurt and gut function.," *American Journal of Clinical Nutrition,* vol. 80, no. 2, pp. 245-56, 2004.

[234] H. Tomotake, "Comparison between Holstein cow's milk and Japanese-Saanen goat's milk in fatty acid composition, lipid digestibility and protein profile.," *Bioscience, Biotechnology and Biochemistry,* vol. 70, no. 11, pp. 2771-2774, 2006.

[235] The University of Granada, "https://www.sciencedaily.com/releases/2007/07/070730100229.htm," *Science Daily,* 31 July 2007.

[236] S. Naaz, "19 Amazing Health Benefits of Mussels," 20 September 2017. [Online]. Available: http://www.stylecraze.com/articles/amazing-health-benefits-of-mussels/#gref. [Accessed 18 December 2017].

[237] Food Allergy Research & Resource Programme, "Molluscan shellfish," 10 March 2014. [Online]. Available: https://farrp.unl.edu/informallmollshellfish. [Accessed 28 November 2017].

[238] University of Manchester Faculty of Biology, Medicine and Health, "Allergy Information for Squid," 18 October 2006. [Online]. Available: http://research.bmh.manchester.ac.uk/informall/allergenic-food/?FoodId=5009. [Accessed 3 December 2017].

[239] L. Mathieu, "the History of Mustard in France," 2017. [Online]. Available: https://www.thegoodlifefrance.com/the-history-of-mustard-in-france/. [Accessed 18 December 2017].

[240] the Telegraph Food, "National Mustard day: 12 fascinating facts about the condiment," 31 July 2015. [Online]. Available: http://www.telegraph.co.uk/foodanddrink/11774083/12-fascinating-facts-about-mustard.html. [Accessed 23 December 2017].

[241] J. Figueroa, "Mustard allergy confirmed by double-blind placebo-controlled food challenges: clinical features and cross-reactivity with mugwort pollen and plant-derived foods.," *Allergy,* vol. 60, no. 1, pp. 48-55, 2005.

[242] L. Leemans, "Consumer study on the use of patient information leaflets," *Journal de Pharmacie de Belgique,* vol. 12, no. 4, pp. 109-116, 2011.

[243] K. Brownell, "The Trans-Fat Ban — Food Regulation and Long-Term Health," *The New England Journal of Medicine,* vol. 370, pp. 1773-1775, 2014.

[244] European Parliament Briefing, "Trans Fats - Overview of Recent Developments," March 2016. [Online]. Available: http://www.europarl.europa.eu/RegData/etudes/BRIE/2016/577966/EPRS_BRI(2016)577966_EN.pdf. [Accessed 30 November 2017].

[245] A. Tammarro, "Magnesium stearate: an underestimated allergen.," *Journal of Biological Regulators and Homeostatic Agents,* vol. 26, no. 4, pp. 783-4, 2012.

[246] European Medicines Agency, "Questions and answers on wheat starch containing gluten in the context of the revision of the guideline on 'Excipients in the label and package leaflet of medicinal products for human use' (CPMP/463/00 Rev. 1)," 24 July 2014. [Online]. Available: http://www.ema.europa.eu/docs/en_GB/document_library/Scientific_guideline/2014/08/WC500170476.pdf. [Accessed 2 December 2017].

[247] Coeliac UK, "Medication, Hospital Visits and Vaccinations," [Online]. Available: https://www.coeliac.org.uk/coeliac-disease/medications-and-vaccinations/. [Accessed 2 December 2017].

[248] J. Robles, "Hypersensitivity Reaction After Inhalation of a Lactose-Containing Dry Powder Inhaler," *Journal of Paediatric Pharmacology and Therapeutics,* vol. 19, no. 3, pp. 206-211, 2014.

[249] W. Klaringbold, "Kinetics and retention of solanidine in man," *Xenobiotica,* vol. 12, no. 5, pp. 293-302, 2012.

[250] T. Mensinga, "Potato glycoalkaloids and adverse effects in humans: an ascending dose study," *Regulatory Toxicology and Pharmacology,* vol. 41, no. 1, pp. 66-72, 2005.

[251] T. Kuiper-Goodman, "Solanine and Chaconine," 1992. [Online]. Available: http://www.inchem.org/documents/jecfa/jecmono/v30je19.htm. [Accessed 2 December 2017].

[252] S. Rodriguez-Stanley, "The effects of capsaicin on reflux, gastric emptying and dyspepsia.," *Alimentary Pharmacology & Therapeutics,* vol. 14, no. 1, pp. 129-134, 2000.

[253] N. Childres, "An Apparent Relation of Nightshades (Solanaceae) to Arthritis," *Journal of Neurological and Orthopedic Medical Surgery,* vol. 12, pp. 227-231, 1993.

[254] J. Prousky, "The use of Niacinamide and Solanaceae (Nightshade) Elimination in the Treatment of Osteoarthritis," *Journal of Orthomolecular Medicine,* vol. 30, no. 1, pp. 13-21, 2015.

[255] A. Fasano, "Leaky gut and autoimmune diseases.," *Clinical Reviews in Allergy & Immunology,* vol. 42, no. 1, pp. 71-78, 2012.

[256] S. Croco, "Potato sprouts and greening potatoes: Potential toxic reaction.," 1981. [Online]. Available: ttps://www.accessdata.fda.gov/scripts/Plantox/Detail.CFM?ID=6537. [Accessed 2 December 2017].

[257] B. Patel, "Potato glycoalkaloids adversely affect intestinal permeability and aggravate inflammatory bowel disease.," *Inflammatory Bowel Diseases,* vol. 8, no. 5, pp. 340-346, 2002.

[258] E. Jensen-Jarolim, "Hot spices influence permeability of human intestinal epithelial monolayers.," *The Journal of Nutrition,* vol. 128, no. 3, pp. 577-581, 1998.

[259] S. Ayad, "Effect of Solanine on Arthritis Symptoms in Postmenopausal Female," *Arab Journal of Nuclear Science and Applications,* vol. 46, no. 3, pp. 279-285, 2013.

[260] J. Ramsey, "Potato History," [Online]. Available: https://www.best-potato-recipes.com/potato-history.html. [Accessed 18 December 2017].

[261] The International Potato Centre, "Potato," 2017. [Online]. Available: https://cipotato.org/crops/potato/. [Accessed 23 December 2017].

[262] GreatBritishChefs, "Know Your Spuds: Our Ultimate Potato Guide," 26 November 2015. [Online]. Available: http://www.greatbritishchefs.com/features/potato-variety-guide. [Accessed 23 December 2017].

[263] G. Mateljan, "The World's Healthiest Foods - Potatoes," 2017. [Online]. Available: http://www.whfoods.com/genpage.php?tname=foodspice&dbid=48. [Accessed 2 December 2017].

[264] J. Wong, "Colonic health: fermentation and short chain fatty acids.," *Journal of Clinical Gastroenterology,* vol. 40, no. 3, pp. 235-243, 2006.

[265] V. Lablokov, "Naturally occurring glycoalkaloids in potatoes aggravate intestinal inflammation in two mouse models of inflammatory bowel disease.," *Digestive Diseases and Sciences,* vol. 55, no. 11, pp. 1158-9, 2010.

[266] M. Cantwell, "A Review of Important Facts about Potato Glycoalkaloids," *Perishables Handling Newsletter,* no. 87, p. 26, 1996.

[267] N. Nahar, "Transcript profiling of two potato cultivars during glycoalkaloid-inducing treatments shows differential expression of genes in sterol and glycoalkaloid metabolism," *Nature: Scientific Reports,* vol. 7, 2017.

[268] K. Smith, "why the Tomato Was Feared in Europe for More Than 200 Years," *Smithsonian Magazine,* 18 June 2013.

[269] J. Cooperstone, "Tomatoes protect against development of UV-induced keratinocyte carcinoma via metabolomic alterations.," *Scientific Reports,* vol. 7, no. 1, p. 5106, 2017.

[270] T. Boileau, "Prostate carcinogenesis in N-methyl-N-nitrosourea (NMU)-testosterone-treated rats fed tomato powder, lycopene, or energy-restricted diets.," *Journal of the National Cancer Institute,* vol. 95, no. 21, pp. 1578-1586, 2003.

[271] M. Friedman, "Tomatine-containing green tomato extracts inhibit growth of human breast, colon, liver, and stomach cancer cells.," *The Journal of Agricultural and Food Chemistry,* vol. 57, no. 13, pp. 5727-33, 2009.

[272] P. Palozza, "Tomato Lycopene and Inflammatory Cascade: Basic Interactions and Clinical Implications," *Current Medicinal Chemistry,* vol. 17, no. 23, pp. 2547-2563, 2010.

[273] G. Mateljan, "The World's Healthiest Foods: Tomatoes," 2017. [Online]. Available: http://www.whfoods.com/genpage.php?tname=foodspice&dbid=44. [Accessed 18 December 2017].

[274] G. Mateljan, "Eggplant," 2017. [Online]. Available: http://whfoods.org/genpage.php?tname=foodspice&dbid=22#healthb enefits. [Accessed 18 December 2017].

[275] P. Capriles, "Effect of eggplant (Solanum melongena) extract on the in vitro labeling of blood elements with technetium-99m and on the biodistribution of sodium pertechnetate in rats.," *Cellular and Molecular Biology,* vol. 48, no. 7, pp. 771-776.

[276] P. Jorge, "Effect of eggplant on plasma lipid levels, lipidic peroxidation and reversion of endothelial dysfunction in experimental hypercholesterolemia," *Arquivos Brasileiros de Cardiologia,* vol. 70, no. 2, pp. 87-91, 1998.

[277] R. Lo Scalzo, "Thermal treatment of eggplant (Solanum melongena L.) increases the antioxidant content and the inhibitory effect on human neutrophil burst.," *Journal of Agricultural and Food Chemistry,* vol. 58, no. 6, pp. 3371-3379, 2010.

[278] B. Babu, "Clinico-Immunological Analysis of Eggplant (Solanum melongena) Allergy Indicates Preponderance of Allergens in the Peel.," *The World Allergy Organization Journal,* vol. 2, no. 9, pp. 192-200, 2009.

[279] G. Mateljan, "World's Healthiest Foods: Bell Peppers," 2017. [Online]. Available: http://whfoods.org/genpage.php?tname=foodspice&dbid=50. [Accessed 18 December 2017].

[280] G. Mateljan, "The Words Healthiest Foods: Bell Pepper," 2017. [Online]. Available: http://whfoods.org/genpage.php?tname=foodspice&dbid=50. [Accessed 18 December 2017].

[281] J. Braaten, "Oat beta-glucan reduces blood cholesterol concentration in hypercholesterolemic subjects.," *European Journal of Clinical Nutrition,* vol. 48, no. 7, pp. 465-474, 1994.

[282] A. Jenkins, "Depression of the glycemic index by high levels of β-glucan fiber in two functional foods tested in type 2 diabetes," *European Journal of Clinical Nutrition,* vol. 56, p. 622–628, 2002.

[283] A. Regand, "The molecular weight, solubility and viscosity of oat beta-glucan affect human glycemic response by modifying starch digestibility," *Food Chemistry,* vol. 129, no. 2, pp. 297-304, 2011.

[284] G. Mateljan, "Brown Rice," 11 December 2017. [Online]. Available: http://www.whfoods.com/genpage.php?tname=foodspice&dbid=128. [Accessed 16 December 2017].

[285] Y. Jeon, "Identification of major rice allergen and their clinical significance in children," *Korean Journal of Pediatrics,* vol. 54, no. 10, p. 414–421, 2011.

[286] P. Williams, "Greatly enhanced arsenic shoot assimilation in rice leads to elevated grain levels compared to wheat and barley," *Environmental Science & Technology,* vol. 41, no. 19, pp. 6854-6859, 2007.

[287] E. Sohn, "Contamination: The toxic side of rice," *Nature,* p. S62– S63, 30 October 2014.

[288] Y. Wei, "Rice consumption and urinary concentrations of arsenic in US adults," *International Journal of Environmental Health Research,* vol. 24, no. 5, pp. 459-470, 2014.

[289] A. Meharg, "Inorganic arsenic levels in rice milk exceed EU and US drinking water standards.," *Journal of Environmental Monitoring,* vol. 10, no. 4, pp. 428-431, 2008.

[290] M. Jung, "Inorganic arsenic contents in ready-to-eat rice products and various Korean rice determined by a highly sensitive gas chromatography-tandem mass spectrometry.," *Food Chemistry,* vol. 1, no. 240, pp. 1179-1183, 2018.

[291] S. Tapio, "Arsenic in the aetiology of cancer," *Mutation Research,* vol. 612, no. 3, pp. 215-46, 2006.

[292] S. Chen, "Elevated risk of hypertension induced by arsenic exposure in Taiwanese rural residents: possible effects of manganese superoxide dismutase (MnSOD) and 8-oxoguanine DNA glycosylase (OGG1) genes.," *Archives of Toxicology,* vol. 86, no. 6, pp. 869-878, 2012.

[293] C. Chen, "Arsenic and diabetes and hypertension in human populations: a review.," *Toxicology and Applied Pharmacology,* vol. 222, no. 3, pp. 298-304, 2007.

[294] P. Balakumar, "Arsenic exposure and cardiovascular disorders: an overview," *Cardiovascular Toxicology,* vol. 9, no. 4, pp. 169-176, 2009.

[295] A. Vahidnia, "Arsenic neurotoxicity--a review," *Human & Experimental Toxicology,* vol. 26, no. 10, pp. 823-832, 2007.

[296] M. Sengupta, "Arsenic burden of cooked rice: Traditional and modern methods.," *Food and Chemical Toxicology,* vol. 44, no. 11, pp. 1823-1829, 2006.

[297] A. Raab, "Cooking rice in a high water to rice ratio reduces inorganic arsenic content.," *Journal of Environmental Monitoring,* vol. 11, no. 1, pp. 41-44, 2009.

[298] Food Standards Authority, "Arsenic in Rice," 25 February 2016. [Online]. Available: https://www.food.gov.uk/science/arsenic-in-rice. [Accessed 16 December 2017].

[299] I. Skypala, "Sensitivity to food additives, vaso-active amines and salicylates: a review of the evidence.," *Clinical and Translational Allergy,* vol. 5, no. 34, 2015.

[300] T. Werfel, "Skin manifestations in food allergy," *Allergy,* vol. 56, no. Suppl 67, pp. 98-101, 2001.

[301] F. Cardinale, "Intolerance to food additives: an update," *Minerva Pediatrica,* vol. 60, no. 6, pp. 1401-1409, 2008.

[302] A. Swain, "Salicylates in foods," *Journal of the American Dietetic Association,* vol. 85, no. 8, pp. 950-960, 1985.

[303] M. Waseem, "Salicylate Toxicity," 21 December 2016. [Online]. Available: https://emedicine.medscape.com/article/1009987-overview. [Accessed 15 December 2017].

[304] S. Sicherer, "Prevalence of peanut and tree nut allergy in the US determined by a random digit dial telephone survey.," *Journal of Allergy and Clinical Immunology,* vol. 103, no. 4, pp. 559-62, 1999.

[305] S. Sicherer, "Peanut and soy allergy: a clinical and therapeutic dilemma," *European Journal of Allergy and Clinical Immunology,* vol. 55, no. 6, pp. 515-521, 2000.

[306] G. Mateljan, "Sesame Seeds," 2017. [Online]. Available: http://whfoods.org/genpage.php?tname=foodspice&dbid=84. [Accessed 5 December 2017].

[307] J. Anderson, "Soy protein effects on serum lipoproteins: a quality assessment and meta-analysis of randomized, controlled studies," *Journal of the American College of Nutrition,* vol. 30, no. 2, pp. 79-91, 2011.

[308] L. Butler, "A vegetable-fruit-soy dietary pattern protects against breast cancer among postmenopausal Singapore Chinese women," *The American Journal of Clinical Nutrition,* vol. 91, no. 4, p. 1013–1019, 2010.

[309] D. Yimit, "Effects of soybean peptide on immune function, brain function, and neurochemistry in healthy volunteers.," *Nutrition,* vol. 28, no. 2, pp. 154-9, 2012.

[310] H. Patisaul, "The pros and cons of phytoestrogens.," *Frontiers in Neuroendocrinology,* vol. 31, no. 4, pp. 400-419, 2010.

[311] American College of Allergy, Asthma and Immunology, "Soy Allergy," 2014. [Online]. Available: http://acaai.org/allergies/types/food-allergies/types-food-allergy/soy-allergy. [Accessed 5 December 2017].

[312] Food Allergy Research and Resource Programme, "Soybeans and Soy Lecithin," April 2017. [Online]. Available: https://farrp.unl.edu/soy-lecithin. [Accessed 5 December 2017].

[313] E. Ros, "Health Benefits of Nut Consumption," *Nutrients,* vol. 2, no. 7, p. 652–682, 2010.

[314] M. Liu, "Tree nut allergy: risk factors for development, mitigation of reaction risk and current efforts in desensitization.," *Expert Review of Clinical Immunology,* vol. 11, no. 5, pp. 673-679, 2015.

[315] J. Van der Valk, "Systematic review on cashew nut allergy," *Allergy,* vol. 69, no. 6, pp. 692-698, 2014.

[316] G. Zhang, "Prevalence of Salmonella in Cashews, Hazelnuts, Macadamia Nuts, Pecans, Pine Nuts, and Walnuts in the United States.," *Journal of Food Protection,* vol. 80, no. 3, pp. 459-466, 2017.

[317] A. Byrne, "How do we know when peanut and tree nut allergy have resolved, and how do we keep it resolved?," *Clinical and Experimental Allergy: the Journal of the British Society for Allergy and Clinical Immunology,* vol. 40, no. 9, pp. 1303-11, 2010.

[318] J. King, "Tree Nuts and Peanuts as Components of a Healthy Diet," *The American Society for Nutrition,* vol. 138, no. 9, pp. 1736S-1740S, 2008.

[319] R. Kohlenberg, "Tyramine sensitivity in dietary migraine: a critical review.," *Headache,* vol. 22, no. 1, pp. 30-34, 1992.

[320] J. Van Eaton, "Tyramine-free Diets," 23 May 2017. [Online]. Available: https://www.healthline.com/health/tyramine-free-diets. [Accessed 23 December 2017].

[321] G. D'Andrea, "Pathogenesis of migraine: role of neuromodulators.," *Headache,* vol. 52, no. 7, pp. 1155-1163, 2012.

[322] Health Research Funding.org, "5 Interesting Facts about Yeast," 27 January 2015. [Online]. Available: https://healthresearchfunding.org/5-interesting-facts-yeast/. [Accessed 7 December 2017].

[323] T. Kelesedis, "Efficacy and safety of the probiotic Saccharomyces boulardii for the prevention and therapy of gastrointestinal disorders," *Therapeutic Advances in Gastroenterology,* vol. 5, no. 2, pp. 111-125, 2012.

[324] Nutritiondata.self.com, "Leavening agents, yeast, bakers, active, dry Nutrition Fact and Calories," 2014. [Online]. Available: http://nutritiondata.self.com/facts/baked-products/5130/2. [Accessed 21 December 2017].

[325] P. Hayes, "Irritable Bowel Syndrome: The Role of Food in Pathogenesis and Management," *Gastroenterology and Hepatology,* vol. 10, no. 3, pp. 164-174, 2014.

[326] H. Weingarten, "Food cravings in a college population," *Appetite,* vol. 17, no. 3, pp. 167-175, 1991.

[327] P. Louis, "Diversity, metabolism and microbial ecology of butyrate-producing bacteria from the human large intestine," *FEMS Microbiology Letters,* vol. 294, no. 1, pp. 1-8, 2009.

[328] The Association for Clinical Biochemistry and Laboratory Medicine, "Allergy Testing," 19 October 2011. [Online]. Available: http://labtestsonline.org.uk/understanding/analytes/allergy/tab/sample. [Accessed 21 November 2017].

[329] NHS Choices, "Which Allergy Test?," 16 February 2016. [Online]. Available: https://www.nhs.uk/Livewell/Allergies/Pages/Whichallergytest.aspx. [Accessed 29 November 2017].

[330] Deutsche Gesellschaft fuer Immunologie e.V./German Society for Immunology, "Allergy: Solving The Mystery Of IgE," 9 September 2009. [Online]. Available: www.sciencedaily.com/releases/2009/09/090914111537.html. [Accessed 21 November 2017].

[331] Coeliac UK, "Myths about coeliac disease," [Online]. Available: https://www.coeliac.org.uk/coeliac-disease/myths-about-coeliac-disease/. [Accessed 28 November 2017].

[332] B. Radford, "Does the human body really replace itself every seven years?," *LiveScience,* no. www.livescience.com/33179-does-human-body-replace-cells-seven-years.html, 4 April 2011.

[333] G. Leisman, "Somatosensory Evoked Potential Changes During Muscle Testing," *International Journal of Neuroscience,* vol. 45, no. 1-2, pp. 143-151, 1989.

[334] W. H. Schmitt, "Correlation of Applied Kinesiology Muscle Testing Findings with Serum Immunologobulin Levels for Food Allergies," 7 July 2009. [Online]. Available: http://www.tandfonline.com/doi/abs/10.3109/00207459808986471. [Accessed 27 November 2017].

[335] A. L. Scopp, "An Experimental Evaluation of Kinesiology in Allergy and Deficiency Disease Diagnosis," *Orthomolecular Psychiatry*, vol. 7, no. 2, pp. 137-138, 1978.

[336] F. Suarez, "A comparison of symptoms after the consumption of milk or lactose-hydrolyzed milk by people with self-reported severe lactose intolerance.," *New England Journal of Medicine*, vol. 333, no. 1, pp. 1-4, 1995.

[337] P. Vernia, "Self-reported milk intolerance in irritable bowel syndrome: what should we believe?," *Clinical Nutrition (Edinburgh, Scotland)*, vol. 23, no. 5, pp. 996-1000, 2004.

[338] I. Bjarnason, "The leaky gut of alcoholism: possible route of entry for toxic compounds.," *Lancet*, vol. 1, no. 8370, pp. 179-182, 1984.

[339] M. Peeters, "Test conditions greatly influence permeation," *Gut*, vol. 35, pp. 1404-1408, 1994.

[340] T. Planninz, "Natural Enzymes to Help Digest Food," 14 August 2017. [Online]. Available: https://www.livestrong.com/article/262840-what-fruits-contain-protease-enzymes/. [Accessed 5 December 2017].

[341] F. Yang, "Studies on germination conditions and antioxidant contents of wheat grain," *International Journal of Food Sciences and Nutrition*, vol. 52, no. 4, pp. 319-330, 2001.

[342] U.S. Geological Survey Water Science School, "The Water in You," 2 December 2016. [Online]. Available: https://water.usgs.gov/edu/propertyyou.html. [Accessed 29 December 2017].

[343] T. Conner, "On carrots and curiosity: Eating fruit and vegetables is associated with greater flourishing in daily life," *British Journal of Health Psychology*, vol. 20, no. 2, p. 413–427, 2015.

[344] L. J, "Health effects of vegetables and fruit: assessing mechanisms of action in human experimental studies1,2,3," *American Society for Clinical Nutrition*, vol. 70, no. 3, pp. 475s-490s, 1999.

[345] J. Chang, "Anal Health Care Basics," *the Permanente Journal,* vol. 20, no. 4, p. 74–80, 2016.

[346] DEFRA, Department of Environment, Food and Rural Affairs, "Dietary Health," in *Food Statistics Pocket Book,* York, 2016, p. 43.

[347] D. Aune, "Fruit and vegetable intake and the risk of cardiovascular disease, total cancer and all-cause mortality—a systematic review and dose-response meta-analysis of prospective studies," *International Journal of Epidemiology,* vol. 46, no. 3, p. 1029–1056, 2017.

[348] A. Drewnowski, "Bitter taste, phytonutrients, and the consumer: a review1,2,3," *American Society for Clinical Nutrition,* vol. 72, no. 6, pp. 1424-1435, 2000.

[349] European Society of Neurogastroenterology and Motility, "Gut Microbiota for Health," 2016. [Online]. Available: http://www.gutmicrobiotaforhealth.com/en/about-gut-microbiota-info/. [Accessed 30 November 2017].

[350] J. Bravo, "Ingestion of Lactobacillus strain regulates emotional behavior and central GABA receptor expression in a mouse via the vagus nerve," *Proceedings of the National Academy of Sciences of the United States of America,* vol. 108, no. 38, p. 16050–16055, 2011.

[351] M. Rogers, "The influence of non-steroidal anti-inflammatory drugs on the gut microbiome.," *Clinical Microbiology and Infection,* vol. 22, no. 2, pp. 178.e1-178.e9, 2016.

[352] X. Liang, "Anti-inflammatory drug and gut bacteria have a dynamic interplay," *Science News,* 4 January 2016.

[353] R. Feltman, "The Gut's Microbiome Changes Rapidly with Diet," *Scientific American,* 14 December 2013.

[354] L. David, "Diet rapidly and reproducibly alters the human gut microbiome," *Nature,* vol. 505, no. 7484, pp. 559-563, 2013.

[355] W. Holzapfel, "Introduction to pre- and probiotics," *Food Research International,* vol. 35, no. 2-3, pp. 109-116, 2002.

[356] J. Slavin, "Fiber and Prebiotics: Mechanisms and Health Benefits," *Nutrients,* vol. 5, no. 4, p. 1417–1435, 2013.

[357] G. Mateljan, "World's healthiest foods," 2015. [Online]. Available: http://whfoods.org/sitesearch.php. [Accessed 9 December 2017].

[358] College of Naturopathic Medicine, "What is Naturopathy?," 2017. [Online]. Available: https://www.naturopathy-uk.com/home/home-what-is-naturopathy/. [Accessed 28 November 2017].

[359] Anaphylaxis.org.uk, "Lupin-allergy-factsheet-july-2016.pdf," July 2016. [Online]. Available: https://www.anaphylaxis.org.uk/wp-content/uploads/2015/06/Lupin-allergy-factsheet-July-2016.pdf. [Accessed 14 November 2017].

[360] J. Buckland, "Eosinophils," [Online]. Available: https://www.immunology.org/public-information/bitesized-immunology/cells/eosinophils. [Accessed 14 November 2017].

[361] A. Lalkhen, "Clinical Tests: Sensitivity and Specificity," *Continuing Education in Anaesthesia Critical Care & Pain,* vol. 8, no. 6, p. 221–223, 1 December 2008.

[362] R. G, "Diagnosing peanut allergy with skin prick and specific IgE testing," *Journal of Allergy and Clinical Immunology,* vol. 115, no. 6, pp. 1291-1296, 2005.

[363] J. Yunginger, "Quantitative IgE antibody assays in allergic diseases," *Journal of Allergy and Clinical Immunology,* vol. 105, no. 6, pp. 1077-1084, 2000.

[364] Food Standards Agency, "Food allergen labelling and information requirements under the EU Food Information for Consumers Regulation No. 1169/2011: Technical Guidance," April 2015. [Online]. Available: https://www.food.gov.uk/sites/default/files/food-allergen-labelling-technical-guidance.pdf. [Accessed 30 November 2017].

[365] T. Ohlsson, "Microwave Technology and Foods," *Advances in food and nutrition Research,* vol. 43, pp. 65-140, 2001.

[366] Z. Yurdagul, "The Differential Diagnosis of Food Intolerance," *Deutsches Artzeblatt International,* vol. 106, no. 21, pp. 359-370, 2009.

[367] J. Tamang, "Functional Properties of Microorganisms in Fermented Foods," *Frontiers in Microbiology,* vol. 7, p. 578, 2016.

[368] L. David, "Diet rapidly and reproducibly alters the human gut microbiome," *Nature,* vol. 505, no. 7484, pp. 559-563, 2014.

[369] S. Shepherd, "Dietary Triggers of Abdominal Symptoms in Patients With Irritable Bowel Syndrome: Randomized Placebo-Controlled Evidence," *Clinical Gastroenterology and Hepatology,* vol. 6, no. 7, pp. 765-771, 2008.

[370] P. Kun-Young, "Health Benefits of Kimchi (Korean Fermented Vegetables) as a Probiotic Food," *Journal of Medicinal Food,* vol. 17, no. 1, pp. 6-20, 2014.

[371] S. Berciano, "Behavior related genes, dietary preferences and anthropometric traits," *Food and Behaviour Research,* vol. 31, no. 1, p. Supplement 299.1, 2017.

[372] R. Heaney, "Calcium absorption in women: relationships to calcium intake, estrogen status, and age.," *Journal of Bone and Mineral Research,* vol. 4, no. 4, pp. 469-75, 1989.

CPSIA information can be obtained
at www.ICGtesting.com
Printed in the USA
LVHW080244181022
730949LV00013B/854